Living with Cancer

Living with Cancer

symptoms ◆ diagnosis ◆ treatment

Dr Jeffrey Tobias and Kay Eaton

BLOOMSBURY

First published in Great Britain in 2001 by
Bloomsbury Publishing Plc
38 Soho Square, London W1D 3HB

By arrangement with the BBC

The BBC logo is a trademark of the British Broadcasting Corporation
and is used under licence.

BBC logo © BBC 1996

A CIP record for this book is available from the British Library.

ISBN 0 7475 5410 2

10 9 8 7 6 5 4 3 2 1

Colour separation by Sang Choy International Pte Ltd, Hong Kong
Printed by Graficromo, Spain

Designed by Alison Shackleton
Edited by Emma Callery
Indexed by Hilary Bird
Illustrations by Anthony Duke

Photographs of Glen Xavier (page 12) and all the patients featured in the
BBC TV series *Living with Cancer* © 2001 BBC/Jon Hall

CONTENTS

FOREWORD

I was delighted when Jeffrey Tobias told me that BBC TV were planning a series about cancer treatment since our son, George, now nine, developed leukaemia just a few weeks after he was born. Michelle and I will never forget the dreadful shock of hearing the diagnosis, at the worst possible time for a young couple just starting a family, and the near-impossibility of coming to terms with what, at the time, felt so totally unbearable.

It seemed as if the bottom had fallen out of our world, but happily and with the fantastic skills of the experts, George's leukaemia turned out to be completely curable. We all know that others are not always so lucky, even though seven out of every ten children now diagnosed with cancer are, like George, totally cured.

I was also very pleased when Dr Tobias asked if I would supply a brief introduction for this book. I've been involved with the BBC for longer than I care to remember, and in any event, I've known him for some years now, since we're both closely involved with a children's cancer charity, raising funds for equipment at the UCL Hospitals Group in London, where the TV series was filmed. I also welcomed the opportunity not only to underline the ever-increasing reality of cure but, in addition, to point out the importance of teamwork and professionalism essential for achieving the best possible result. A parent is probably better placed than anybody to see this at first hand – not just the doctors and nurses on the wards, but also the pharmacists, physiotherapists, play specialists, dieticians, radiographers operating the radiotherapy machines... the list is almost endless. To use a footballing analogy, it may be the Beckhams and Owens who score the goals but none of it would happen without the skills of the guys at the back, the coaches on the benches and the largely invisible club staff behind the scenes who keep the whole thing moving.

This book covers a lot of ground, giving information about diagnosis and treatment, and also, though space is obviously limited, dealing with the psychological issues raised by a diagnosis of cancer. Jeff Tobias and Kay Eaton are very well placed to do this, and have blended together essential information which is difficult for the non-specialist to get hold of from other sources. They've also described, by direct interviews with patients appearing in the series, the human side of coping with the diagnosis and treatment, warts and all. Obviously it can't always make happy reading, particularly since we have still so far to go with so many cancers currently resistant to treatment. I know of course that my own experience with cancer in the family has had a happier out-come than for many others, but real advances are being made all the time, as both the book and the TV series reveal. Everyone stands to benefit from more access to facts and explanation, particularly since malignant diseases are now so common that most individuals and families will have at least a passing acquain-tance.

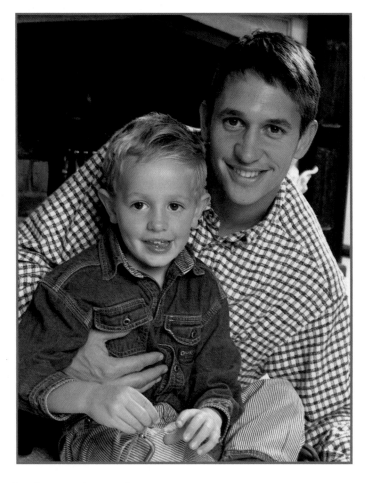

We all hope this book will help in that aim, providing useful information and support and hopefully going some way towards demystifying such a frightening illness. Jeff, Kay and I are grateful to BBC TV for their enthusiasm and commitment, to the Cancer Research Campaign for help with facts and figures, and finally to all the patients and hospital staff involved in the series.

GARY LINEKER

INTRODUCTION

Over the past 50 years, the incidence of cancer has risen steadily, to the point where it is now diagnosed in about a quarter of a million people in the UK each year. Although it causes one in four of all deaths, many in younger people, the good news is that over recent years, cancer treatment has dramatically improved as well, for almost all cancers both the common and the rare. For example, the past decade has seen a remarkable decline in breast cancer deaths, down 30% in middle-aged women as a result of better treatment. In testicular cancer, over a slightly longer time interval, the death rate has been cut even more dramatically, by 70 per cent.

It may come as a surprise to many that for quite a large number of patients, cancer is readily curable, with few if any consequences. Patients with the more common types of skin cancer are almost always curable by surgery, radiotherapy or other form of treatment. Even in men with melanoma, which is the most malignant of skin tumours, the five-year survival (frequently regarded as the key statistic in cancer) improved from 46% (1971–75) to 68% (1986–90) – a remarkable increase of 22%.

For some types of cancer, including leukaemia, chemotherapy has become the cornerstone of treatment and surgery has little if any part to play, whereas for others, the best approach to cure may well be through the use of radiotherapy – certain cancers of the head and neck, for example, where a very high cure rate plus preservation of normal function can be achieved by radiotherapy. Many patients with cancer of the larynx, for example, fall into this category.

There are many types of cancer with a five-year survival rate over 50% but overall survival rates are nowhere near as good as this – largely because of the very high incidence of lung cancer, one of the most common, lethal and yet most preventable types of cancer in adults, responsible for almost 35,000 deaths in the UK each year. In the 1950s, the male:female ratio was 6:1 but with the much increased frequency of smoking in women, female lung cancer cases have shot up as well, to 24,000 new cases annually in men and 14,500 in women (1997 figures). The next most common cancers, breast and bowel, have a much better outlook – as outlined further on in the book. In children, cancer is sadly the most common cause of 'natural' death, exceeded only by deaths from injury and road traffic accidents. But in this age group improvements in outlook have been astonishing, with over seven cures out of every ten children diagnosed with cancer.

UNDERSTANDING CANCER

We've written this book to accompany the BBC TV series *Living with Cancer*. The idea of providing what we hope will be an informative, practical and supportive guide seemed too good to miss, particularly since our work in one of London's largest cancer centres brings us face-to-face with so many patients, and we're all too aware of the misconceptions and lack of information which so many patients, friends and family complain about. All too often, people's perception of the illness and its treatment is seriously wide of the mark – not surprising, perhaps, since cancer medicine moves at a remarkable rate. New treatments, often in their most preliminary stage, are increasingly pounced upon by the media, almost before the ink is dry on the first research paper.

We know quite a lot about the causes of cancer. In Victorian times, relatively few people died of it – partly because many died younger of other causes. Now it is responsible for over 150,000 deaths in the UK each year, not only due to our ever-increasing lifespan, but for additional reasons relating to lifestyle. The enormous rise in smoking, which became seriously popular at about the time of the First World War, caused not only a huge increase in lung cancer, but many other types as well: mouth, lip, larynx, kidney, bladder, pancreas, cervix and so on. Obesity has now been recognised as another key factor, probably playing an important part in the development of 10 to 15% of all cancers. Our quest for 'healthy' tans and our love of sunbathing has led to a huge increase in the rates of skin cancer. By the year 2020 it is expected that malignant melanoma, much the most serious form of skin cancer which doesn't yet feature in the 'top 10' in cancer mortality in the UK, will have risen sharply, up to ninth position.

Other predictions are that with a decline in smoking, improvements in treatment and diet, and possibly new preventive drugs, lung cancer – currently at number one position - will have fallen to fourth place, over-taken by prostate, breast and bowel cancers; whereas bladder, stomach, lymphoma and oesophagus, currently occupying positions five to nine, will remain more or less unchanged, though the incidence of oesophageal cancer is rising sharply. Cancer of the cervix is essentially the result of viral infection and has been virtually eradicated in some Nordic countries, through highly successful screening programmes. But in the developing world, with little in the way of screening and an increasingly unhealthy Western-dominated lifestyle (more cigarette smoking, heavy drinking, too much red meat, too little fibre and not enough exercise), then the rates are bound to rise sharply.

We were delighted when the BBC responded to our suggestion for a TV series that would chronicle the lives of patients undergoing treatment for newly-diagnosed cancer, both to try and break down some of the taboos that surround this disease as no other, and also to show how much can be done to help, and wherever possible provide a cure. Although cancer touches the lives of so many of us, few people really understand what radiotherapy and chemotherapy, for example, are all about. Many think of these as appalling and damaging treatments with little if any benefit for the patient, rather than – as in our view – treatments, which despite the danger of possible side-effects, can transform patients' lives and often provide a cure. One of the aims of this book – and indeed the TV series it accompanies – is to try to explain in sensible language both the key features of various types of cancer and also to describe the range of treatments available, and the extraordinary expertise of the many talented professionals whose skills are so vital.

ABOUT THIS BOOK

Approximately one third the book covers cancer-related topics of general interest: causes, genetic predisposition, the sometimes baffling differences in cancer prevalence in various parts of the world, and so on. The rest of the book covers the specific cancers in more detail, with the emphasis on the most common types, their different patterns of behaviour and for each one, an account of the main approaches to treatment. Through lack of space, some of the newer areas of cancer research can't be covered in full detail. But what we set out to do is to try and demystify first of all the subject itself, both the general issues relating to cancer and also some of the specifics; and in addition to empower patients as much as possible. The word 'cancer' still carries far too many of the traditional connotations, despite the increased openness with which we now discuss it. Wherever possible, we're keen to dispel the often persisting sense of helplessness and shock, and replace it by a message of hope and optimism. More and more patients are now cured, treatment side-effects are being reduced, cancer pain and other symptoms have become far more controllable. Patients with cancer usually live highly active lives, in many cases even after the cancer has spread to other parts of the body, and a full cure has become impossible.

Contributions from patients – several of whom are featured in the TV series – form an extremely important part of this book. We interviewed as many as possible, to try to get to the heart of their perception and experience of the illness. No one could give a clearer account of this than the person who has been through it for him- (or her)self. For the staff in the hospital – not just doctors and nursing staff, but radiographers, pharmacists, physiotherapists, social workers and so many more – the opportunity to talk to patients, as well as providing their own skilled professional help, provides the most gratifying part of all that we do. We won't pretend that the resources for cancer treatment are all we would wish; in many parts of the country, the provision of radiotherapy equipment, for example, is clearly inadequate and waiting lists far too long. But an additional injection of government funds has already started to improve the situation and more and more treatment centres now co-operate with each other, forming 'cancer networks', which should ensure higher standards. In some cases, for example breast cancer, survival figures have risen quite remarkably over the past decade, partly through screening, but more importantly through dramatic improvements in treatment which look set to continue.

As well as the patient contributions that thread through the book, we've deliberately provided a lengthy section in the form of questions and answers – the most commonly asked questions that patients put to us with, we hope, honest and straightforward answers. Needless to say, this book doesn't pretend to be a comprehensive cancer text, but we hope it will prove helpful and informative.

OUR THANKS

We're extremely grateful to Gary Lineker, who's already done so much to raise funds for cancer treatment, for providing the perfect personal introduction, and to the Cancer Research Campaign for financial and statistical support.

Even more, we wish to thank the patients and all the staff at University College London NHS Hospitals Trust, who have all been unswerving in their support for both the TV series and the book. Every department in the hospital has been involved in one way or another –

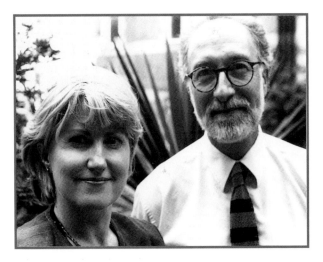

most particularly, of course, the Meyerstein Institute of Oncology, and the Departments of Medicine, Surgery and Haematology to whom we extend our particular thanks. Staff and patients alike have been endlessly patient, but the task was made so much easier by the great sensitivity of the BBC production staff, especially Emma Hindley, Charlotte Moore, Sam Bickley, Miriam Jones and Kerry Ranscombe. We'd also like to thank Julie Sheppard from the UCLH Press and Public Relations Department, and to acknowledge the critical input of Paul Hamann, who was Head of Documentaries at the BBC when we first suggested the idea for a TV cancer series. Jenny Abbott, the BBC's Executive Producer, Nicky Thompson and Kathy Rooney from Bloomsbury have all been warmly supportive and provided ideas, common-sense and imaginative suggestions in equal measure. Sue Osborne and Gordon McVie have been our key contacts at the Cancer Research Campaign. Although the CRC supplied many of the facts and figures that illustrate the book, any errors are strictly our own responsibility.

Finally, we would like to dedicate the book to the hundreds of highly skilled staff at the hospital, whose commitment and professionalism ensure that all our patients receive the best possible standards of care.

JEFFREY TOBIAS AND KAY EATON

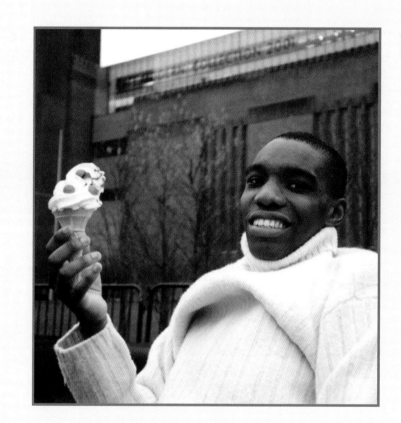

PART ONE

THE FACTS ABOUT CANCER

' Day to day I try not to focus on what my disease is doing. I'd rather focus on what my life's doing and then find out where the disease fits inside that – otherwise you become preoccupied with just living to die rather than the other way. '

GLEN XAVIER

WHO GETS CANCER? WHY ME?

what we know about the causes of cancer

Within the past year or two, cancer has outstripped heart attack and other cardiovascular disorders as the leading cause of death in the UK. Paradoxically, cancer deaths continue to fall here, but deaths from heart disease have fallen at a faster rate. In the 50 years between 1950 and 1999, cancer deaths rose from 15% to 27% of total deaths (men) and from 16% to 23% (women). As cancer is largely a disease of the elderly, and we're generally living longer now, these figures will probably rise further. Two-thirds of all cancers occur over the age of 65 years.

In many types of cancer we have little or no idea what might have triggered the initial malignant change. Just as with known potential causes of heart disease – high blood pressure, lack of exercise, the wrong kind of food and so on – cancer is clearly a multifactorial illness in terms of its causes or origins. Even more baffling is the curious chain of events that might lead a cancer to spread from its initial position in the body (the 'primary site'), leading to more distant secondary tumours. We do, however, have many clues, mostly in the form of cancer genetics, studies of different populations throughout the world (epidemiology), and the chain of events leading towards malignant change (cancer carcinogenesis). We now recognise that although over 200,000 people develop cancer in the UK each year, mostly during the second half of their lives, a few cancers predominate. Cancers of the lung, breast, prostate and lower bowel (colorectal) account for over half of all cases. Each has a different causation, and the main points are outlined below.

SMOKING

Age-standardised mortality, the major causes of death in England and Wales between 1950 and 1999.

Lung cancer is numerically the most important of all at 16% of all new cancer cases and we've known for years how to dramatically reduce its frequency. About 50% of all smokers will die prematurely as a result of

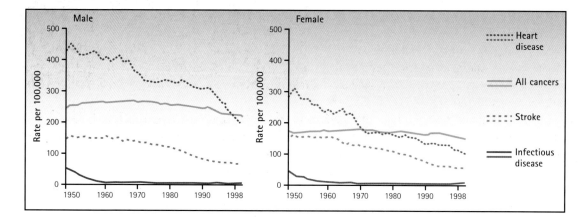

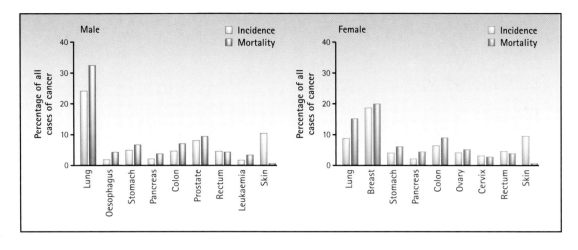

Incidence and mortality of cancer in the United Kingdom.

cigarettes, or 500 out of every 1000 compared with one from criminal violence and six or seven from accidents.

Lung cancer is a particularly fascinating and tragic example of a tumour in which we know almost all we need to know about causation in order to eradicate it altogether (or very nearly); yet this common and often fatal tumour remains the main cause of cancer death in most parts of Europe and the USA. The strength of the data linking cigarette smoking to lung cancer can hardly be over-emphasised, the increased incidence following a sharp rise in cigarette smoking, first in men between the two world wars and more recently in women as well. In the 1950s, the male:female ratio for lung cancer was about ten to one, whereas the figure now is less than three to one, simply as a result of the women catching up. Lung cancer is now common, even in relatively young women in their forties and fifties. However, there's good news too: stopping smoking sharply reduces the risk. After about 12 years, the danger level falls almost as low as for non-smokers. The sad fact is that about half of all smokers die prematurely for one reason or another, chiefly as a result of cancers or heart disease, both of course far more common in people who smoke.

Why do different populations have such widely differing rates of cancer incidence? Some groups smoke more, some less. In the USA, the incidence of lung cancer among professional white males has fallen recently, whereas in other parts of the world, particularly China and the Far East, lung cancer rates continue to rise as smoking becomes more prevalent with little or no attempt at educating the population. In the UK, smoking frequency is largely related to socio-economic class and geography. The greatest risks are in the north of the country (particularly in younger people), with some counties as much as 50-70% above

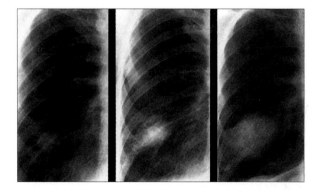

Lung cancer: this tumour grew gradually over a period of 18 months (the patient declined any form of treatment). It is clearly visible as an enlarging mass in the lower lobe of the right lung.

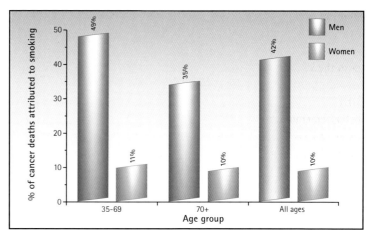

This chart shows the percentage of all cancer deaths attributed to cigarette smoking in developed countries (figures from 1990).

average. London, which had the highest rates before the Second World War, is now about average.

Some agents, such as cigarette smoke, are clearly liable to cause a cancerous change (carcinogenic), but what is it within them that is the real culprit? Is it possible to produce a really safe cigarette by excluding the dangerous chemical? And what about the biological processes that take place within the cell when a cancer change is triggered?

In the case of lung cancer, many of the constituents of cigarette smoke are thought to be carcinogenic, including nicotine itself, trace elements, and toxic, organic chemicals, such as benzpyrene and benzofluoranthenes (they even sound dangerous!). A particularly aggressive form of lung cancer affecting the outer covering, or pleura, of the lung is clearly associated with previous exposure to asbestos. This is dealt with more fully on pages 68-9.

It is also important to note that cigarette smoking doesn't only cause lung cancer. It is clearly linked to cancers of the mouth, voice box (larynx), pancreas, kidney and bladder – these latter two, presumably, because of cigarette smoke carcinogens, which are concentrated in the kidney and held in the bladder before finally leaving the body when the individual urinates. Cancer of the cervix is another tumour in which cigarette smoking appears to be causative. Tobacco used in other ways can also cause cancer to develop. In India, for example, mouth (oral) cancer occurs within the oral cavity, often at a number of sites, due to the widespread habit of retaining a tobacco-betel nut pan in the

ERIC'S STORY

Eric, a retired 74-year-old stockbroker who had stopped smoking ten years ago, initially saw his doctor because of mild shortness of breath and discomfort across the front of the chest. An X-ray showed a 4-centimetre tumour in the left upper lobe with a small cavity within; CT scanning showed no evidence of glandular involvement in the centre of the chest. His general condition was pretty good, so the local chest physician sent him to a thoracic surgeon, who performed his usual pre-operative investigation of walking briskly with the patient up three flights of stairs; he noted that Eric was no more out of breath than he was, and decided he was fit for surgery.

Four years later, after a left upper lobectomy (with preservation of about half of the left lung, leaving the right side untouched), the patient remains well and is probably out of the woods. Even though Eric developed lung cancer from lifelong cigarette smoking, he did himself a great favour by giving up ten years before the diagnosis at the late age of 64 years. His story illustrates the fact that it's never too late to stop smoking – the sooner the better!

mouth throughout the day. Some Third World populations like to smoke with the lit end within the mouth, a potent cause of cancer of the palate. Mouth cancer in India is the common counterpart of lung cancer in the West.

DIET

Diet is emerging as an increasingly important risk factor for lower bowel cancers. We eat far too much fatty processed foods and not enough fruit and vegetables (now recommended as five or more portions daily). For other types of cancer, lifestyle and dietary differences appear to be fairly closely linked with the development of a particular cancer, though the causal relationship is far less clear than with cigarette smoking and lung cancer.

There is a clear relationship between fat intake and the development of breast cancer, and between intake of dietary meat protein and the development of cancer of the large bowel. Yet in each of these cases, is the definable characteristic – the meat in one case, the fat in the other – truly the causative agent? Could it not be that something else about an affluent lifestyle is perhaps the offending initiator of malignant change, with the fat or meat intake simply serving as a marker of, if you like, a too-affluent lifestyle, which departs from some predetermined but more natural dietary state?

AGE

Our risks of developing cancer are also greatly increased as we grow older (see box, right). For breast cancer, aside from genetic (familial) predisposition (see below), important causative factors include age at first pregnancy (the younger the woman is, the less likely she is to develop the cancer), with a three times greater likelihood for women bearing their first child over the age of 30 compared with those under 20 at first pregnancy.

With changing social attitudes, better contraception and increased numbers of women seeking careers, all of which might delay the first pregnancy, this one feature alone could account for the 10% increase in the incidence of breast cancer noted in both the UK and USA in the 1970s and early 1980s. Breast cancer has become so common in the Western world that one in ten women are now expected to develop it at some point during their lifetime, with even greater prevalence in certain parts of the country.

GENETIC PREDISPOSITION

Some families clearly have a genetic predisposition to cancer, with some family members developing cancers of a particular type. Up to 10% of common cancers, particularly those of breast, ovary and large bowel, appear to occur in familial clusters, with a predisposition in these families to a particular inherited gene, with the implication that

---

THE IMPORTANCE OF AGE AS A DISCRIMINATING FACTOR

The incidence of many cancers increases with age. For some cancers, age may be one of the most useful discriminating factors.

• *For several common cancers, 1% or less of cases are diagnosed before 40 years. These include:*
Lung
Oesophagus
Stomach
Pancreas
Colon
Rectum
Prostate
Bladder
Endometrium
Larynx
Myeloma

• *For the following cancers only 3 to 5% of cases are diagnosed before 40 years:*
Breast
Ovary
Kidney
Mouth, lip, pharynx

• *For some cancers, the distribution across adult age groups is more even. These include:*
Cervix
Melanoma
Thyroid
Brain
Sarcoma
Non Hodgkin's Lymphoma

• *Some cancers are most common in younger adults (less than 40 years). These include:*
Testicular cancer
Hodgkin's disease

EVIDENCE FOR THE GENETIC BASIS OF HUMAN CANCER

- Chromosome changes are evident in many cancers.

- Most carcinogens are mutagens.

- Increased risk of cancer in syndromes associated with DNA repair defects.

- Simple recessive or dominant inheritance of cancer.

- Related genetic changes in sporadic and familial cancer.

- The identification of activated proto-oncogenes and inactivated tumour suppressor genes.

INDICATIONS OF GENETIC PREDISPOSITION TO CANCER

- Several cancers of the same type on the same side of the family.

- Cancers occurring at young ages (less than 50 years).

- Cancers of particular types that are known to be associated, e.g. breast and ovarian cancer or large bowel and breast.

- Two or more cases of rare cancers in the same family.

- Multiplicity of primary tumours, e.g. bilateral breast cancer.

children of an affected patient would have a 50% risk. However, because of the multifactorial nature of cancer development mentioned above, not all of these patients develop a malignant tumour as many other factors come into play, including the power or penetrance of the genetic predisposition, and probably on dietary and other lifestyle factors as well.

Little is known of the cellular regulating mechanisms that prevent patients who have a strong genetic predisposition from developing their cancer(s) earlier in life. Think, for example, of the extraordinary phenomenon of lower bowel cancer, a common condition with over 28,000 new cases a year in the United Kingdom, which can generally be cured by surgery if the tumour is detected early enough, without evidence of spread. Scientists have now located the gene that causes bowel cancer, situated on the second main chromosome (out of 23 human pairs), following painstaking work on two substantial families with a history of the disease. The work required collaboration between three major research groups in the United States and Finland, and it is now estimated that the defective gene is carried by one in every 200 people in the Western population, or viewed from a different perspective, up to 250,000 people in Britain alone, making this the most common inherited disorder of all. Within the next few years, this should allow testing of high-risk families on a very large scale, with the prospect either of careful regular screening for people carrying the gene but without evidence of the disease, or possibly early surgery in selected cases. Now that we have relatively straightforward means of direct examination of the whole large bowel using fibre-optic methods (colonoscopy), the careful (and repeated) study of such potential patients is technically possible. The difficulty will be in assessing the relative costs and benefits of such an enormous task.

Very few cancers occur solely as a result of genetic predisposition, but in the rare childhood cancer retinoblastoma, a malignant disease of the eye occurring in very young children, there is a powerful familial component, and the genetics are reasonably well understood (see page 186). The rate of this tumour appears to have doubled over the past 50 years, largely due to affected children surviving and having children themselves, many of whom will then be affected. With modern treatment methods, most of the affected children can be cured without serious loss of vision, since radiotherapy and chemotherapy are often at least as effective as surgery. This success story serves well to illustrate the importance of genetic identification and predisposition, and the number of known cases of genetically linked, common cancers does seem to be growing (see also box, left).

ENVIRONMENTAL FACTORS

In testicular cancer, the rise in incidence over the past 25 years remains largely unexplained. Maybe the fall in the average male sperm count,

THE VALUE OF EPIDEMIOLOGY

Epidemiology is the study of populations, their habits, types of illness, dietary preferences and so on. Studies comparing different cancer rates in different parts of the world or in different socio-economic groups, have been extremely productive in our understanding of the various likely causes. For example, the frequency of the five most common cancers is markedly different in the developed compared with the developing world. Obviously the possibility arises that certain foods, behaviour patterns or other aspects of lifestyle might be responsible for the extraordinary differences that occur, though genetics may also play a part. The frequency of migration we see so often has taught us that resettled populations tend to develop the cancer-risk pattern of their new home, suggesting, perhaps, that genetics may be less important than environmental influences.

Epidemiological studies have been extremely powerful in determining changes of cancer incidence in different countries throughout the 70-year period from the 1930s, when accurate record keeping became established. From these studies, we now know, for example, that breast and testicular cancer are still rising in incidence and that cancer of the stomach is clearly on the decline.

possibly related to environmental factors, could in some way be related.

Occupational exposure to dangerous chemicals should largely be a thing of the past, but in former days, it was an important clue to cancer causation. In 1775, the great Bart's surgeon Sir Percivall Pott noted a very high incidence of skin cancer over the scrotum in chimney sweeps, and it later turned out that some of the more unpleasant constituents of coal tar and soot had a direct effect on these poor lads, who, needless to say, ended up covered from head to foot with the carcinogenic materials, though with a particularly high collection of soot and grease in their pelvic skin. About 100 years later, it was noted that workers in dye factories had an unusually high incidence of bladder cancer. Other occupational groups were later identified as well, including workers in cable and rubber factories (see also box, overleaf).

VIRAL CAUSES

In animals, certain viruses are known to cause cancers, and seem an increasingly likely cause of some of our human cancers as well. In China, for example, where cancer in the area behind the nose (post-nasal space or nasopharynx) is common, there appears to be a very high level of contamination by the Epstein-Barr virus, and closer to home, many cases of cancer of the cervix are thought to be linked to a virus passed on during sexual intercourse.

Women with multiple partners, particularly between the ages of 12 and 20 years, are at relatively high risk, though this certainly isn't the whole story. Occasional cases of husbands and wives (or partners) with, on the one hand, a carcinoma of the penis, and on the other, a cancer of the cervix, have been well documented.

For the most part, however, there is no clear-cut relationship

ESTABLISHED CARCINOGENIC AGENTS THAT ARE AN OCCUPATIONAL HAZARD	
Agent	*Site of cancer*
Aromatic amines	Bladder
Arsenic	Skin, lung
Asbestos	Lung, pleura, peritoneum
Benzene	Bone marrow
Bis (chloromethyl) ether	Lung
Cadmium	Prostate
Chromium	Lung
Ionizing irradiation and all other	Bone marrow sites
Isopropyl alcohol manufacture	Nasal sinuses
Leather goods manufacture	Nasal sinuses
Mustard gas	Larynx, lung
Nickel	Nasal sinuses, lung
Polycyclic hydrocarbons	Skin, lung
UV light	Skin, lip
Vinyl chloride	Liver
Wood dust	Nasal sinuses

between a viral causation and the development of human cancer, though viruses may be able to transform cells in a dangerous way, leading to a lengthy, latent period before tumour development. This would make any link between the initiating virus and the subsequent tumour much more difficult to confirm. Other important areas where viral carcinogenesis is thought likely include Kaposi's sarcoma, the classical skin malignancy seen in so many AIDS patients, primary liver cancer (strongly linked to hepatitis B virus), and also Burkitt's lymphoma, typically a tumour encountered in African children and adolescents.

RADIATION

Radiation, so valuable in the treatment of cancer, is itself carcinogenic. This may seem paradoxical but even at relatively low doses, radiation can damage a cell sufficiently to cause a dangerous mutation, and eventually tumour development within the radiation-exposed area. Although the risk of causing a radiation-induced cancer is certainly one that radiotherapists are well aware of, it is generally very low, especially in comparison with the advantages of radiotherapy in controlling a malignant tumour, which cannot easily be dealt with by other means. The risk is, however, an extremely good reason to be cautious with radiotherapy for non-malignant conditions, such as scar overgrowth in surgical wounds or chronic rheumatic disorders.

Radiotherapy causes damage by producing breaks in strands of DNA (the double-helix genetic material discovered by Watson and Crick and present within the cell nucleus), producing chromosomal abnormalities such as breakage, complete disappearance of part of the chromosomal material and the removal of genetic material from one part of the chromosome to another. Although these changes are normally lethal to a cell, rendering it incapable of causing further trouble, they may occur to a level insufficient to kill the cell, allowing it to mutate at a later stage without the normal cell control mechanisms. It is this uncontrolled cellular growth that is generally regarded as being so dangerous.

Several types of cancer are more common after wide-scale radiation exposure, such as occurred at Hiroshima or Chernobyl. These include thyroid cancer, leukaemia and lymphoma and breast cancer. One fascinating fact for the cancer biologist is that it took 40 years for the excess in breast cancer cases to become apparent after the Hiroshima and Nagasaki bombs in 1945, whereas the other tumour types were picked up much more rapidly. This 'lag period' clearly tells us something about the normal developmental biology of these different tumours. Patients so often ask, 'How long have I had it?' and, in truth, there is no easy answer, since we believe cancer is likely to have developed from a single mutant cell – and when on earth might that have taken place?

The only real clue we have to this is that a single, definable exposure to radiation in Hiroshima in 1945 produced an increase in risk, which was detectable for the first time in the mid-1980s. Does this

THE CANCER PATIENT

One myth that needs to be dispelled is that there is no such thing as the 'cancer personality'. This seems to be a very dangerous concept, implying, apart from any other considerations, that at the end of the day, it was your own fault you got it in the first place! There have certainly been patients who have turned elsewhere for advice, only to be told that 'this sequence of events in your recent life, with stress, loss, inability to come to terms with the grief, etc., etc., is the cause!' These sentiments are quite destructive. Cancer patients may be introverted, outgoing, positive or depressed. They are endlessly varied, as with all other patients, and it is both shallow and mischievous to label them in any particular way. There is no evidence whatsoever that a particular personality type is more liable to develop cancer.

There is, however, the question of why some patients are cured of cancer whereas others, with an apparently identical condition, relapse and may ultimately die from it. One celebrated study divided breast cancer patients into four groups: the denial group (who reacted by pretending that it was happening to somebody else, not them); those who displayed 'fighting spirit' ('I'll beat it – it won't get the better of me'); the stoic acceptors, and finally the 'helpless, hopeless' group. The first two groups did far better than the latter two, and all sorts of psychological explanations were put forward to explain this phenomenon. Just think, though, how difficult it is to change one's personality! If you are a natural stoic acceptor, how can you become a classic 'fighting spirit' type? It's one of those areas where it is doubtful that knowing the results of personality studies will actually do anyone any good.

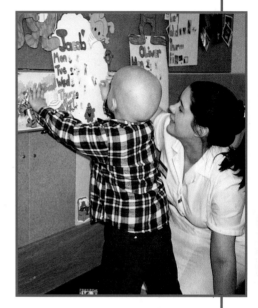

The fact that children are diagnosed with cancer should certainly dispel the myth that there is a 'cancer personality'.

mean that the tumour was in some way slowly developing during this whole period? Probably yes, although the other features of cancer causation would vary – the strength of the family history, for example. Interestingly enough, from our own case records we well remember a patient in her early forties without any past family history of breast cancer, who developed the disease in exactly the same year as her one other sister, a most unlikely coincidence. Further probing of the sisters' histories revealed that their father had contracted TB when they were in their early teens, and as contacts, they had both had an annual chest X-ray for five or six years, a practice that would not now be recommended. This would have been just at the same time as their breasts were developing, and the radiation effect of those multiple repeated chest X-rays might very well have had something to do with the development (in both of them) of a breast cancer within a virtually identical time frame.

WHAT EXACTLY IS CANCER?

Cancer biology is the study of cancer evolution and development at the cellular level. As cancer expert Professor Robert Souhami has written:

'When thinking about cancer, many scientists and physicians, and members of the public, perceive cancer as being "foreign" to the body. Analogies with infections caused by parasites and germs are often drawn, and many infectious agents have been proposed as possible triggers. As knowledge has progressed, however, it has become apparent that, in many respects, cancer cells are similar to normal cells and that there is considerable diversity of function and structure within a single neoplasm (abnormal growth). Even greater diversity exists between tumours of the same type in different individuals and between tumours of different types. The fundamental property of cancer, which distinguishes the disease from normal tissues and which makes treatment so difficult, is metastasis. We are still ignorant of the mechanisms which underlie this remarkable process.'

CANCER IS ESSENTIALLY:
- The disordered and uncontrolled growth of cells within a specific organ or tissue type.
- Most cancers, though not all, begin in a single site, such as breast, lung or brain.
- If left untreated, they grow steadily, often by invading surrounding areas (i.e. growing by direct extension).
- They often also produce secondary growths, often termed 'metastases'. This is the central and most threatening feature of malignant disorders.

The main difficulty in cancer treatment lies in an all-too-frequent failure to deal effectively with these secondary deposits at scattered or distant sites in the body. One of the major reasons why cancer physicians are so obsessed with clinical trials is that so much effort is directed towards protecting patients by means of whole-body treatments, such as chemotherapy or hormones, from the possible development of these life-threatening secondary deposits of tumour.

Although most cancers originate at a single site, this is not always the case. In leukaemia, for example, the malignant transformation of blood or, more accurately, certain elements of the bone marrow (the site of manufacture of specific blood cells), the whole of this tissue is apparently transformed by the single initiating process that triggered the malignant change. Little is known of the causes of human leukaemia, though in animals, for example the domestic cat, a virus is known to be the cause. Blood (or 'haematological') disorders such as leukaemia have a totally different pattern of behaviour from most 'solid' malignancies, though even in the latter, multiple primary tumours do occasionally occur in the same organ, including, for example, the Kaposi sarcoma so prevalent in young men with AIDS.

Despite the single-site origin of most cancers, a second primary (not to be confused with tumour secondaries) can develop in other areas of similar tissue, particularly with cancers of 'paired organs'. For example, patients with breast cancer, though frequently successfully treated, have a higher incidence of a second primary tumour occurring in the opposite breast, possibly as high as 20% over a lengthy follow-up period. Likewise, in testicular tumours, second primary tumours can occur in the opposite testis many years after unequivocal cure at the initial site. Interestingly, one known cause of testicular cancer is the failure of testicular descent at birth, and even though the undescended testicle is at greater risk of malignant change, a definite increased risk is noted in the testis that apparently developed and came down into the scrotal sac quite normally.

In some people, an obvious carcinogen may cause a second primary cancer. Perhaps the most tragic example of this occurs in patients who smoke heavily, develop an early and curable cancer of the larynx – often cured by radiotherapy without any loss of voice or serious side-effect – but then continue to smoke and develop a lung cancer a few years later; a disease with a far worse outlook and higher fatality rate, and all too often incurable.

Cancers not only develop at a single site, but also result from malignant change within a single clone of cells:

• A 'clone' is a cluster of cells derived from a single 'stem' cell.

• This is initiated by a genetic, environmental or other influence (or in most cases, of course, a combination of these), developing into a malignant growth by continued cell division, and producing progeny with the same characteristics and lack of cellular control.

• It is likely that a carcinogenic 'initiator' (the underlying or first event, which destabilises the cell and renders it susceptible to cancer growth) is followed by one or more 'promoter' agents, which produce further transient changes and which eventually cause the cancer to develop.

Several steps are required before a normal cell becomes a malignant one and cell growth and division is profoundly influenced by the presence of critical genes. These fall into two groups: oncogenes, which drive the cell towards malignancy, and suppressor genes, which may mutate and result in a loss of normal regulatory or restraining function. It is often suggested that cellular oncogenes, when activated by carcinogens, initiate the chain of events which leads to malignant transformation.

Oncogenes may be very simply activated, becoming multiplied or 'amplified' within the chromosome, to provide several copies, resulting in relatively rapid malignant development within. With suppressor genes, a greater degree of abnormality – heredity of the abnormality from both parents, for example – may be necessary for the abnormal drive to be powerful enough to initiate malignant change. This may turn out to be highly relevant in breast cancer, since the much-discussed, recently discovered *BRCA-I* and *BRCA-2* genes are thought most likely to be suppressors acting in just this way. The central point is that loss of the tumour-suppressing activity of the critical gene, if present to a sufficient degree, may allow a tumour to develop. The presence and activity of tumour suppressor genes sits comfortably with traditional concepts of 'tumour surveillance', first postulated by Sir Peter Medawar and others 40 years ago. They suggested that we might all be producing potential cancers much of the time, but that most of us have a 'constant-alert' surveillance or scavenging cellular mechanism which recognises these potentially dangerous, early mutational changes and eliminates them before any real damage is done.

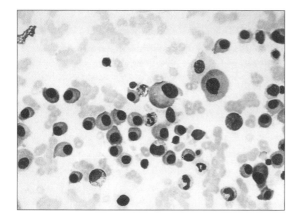

Infiltration of bone marrow with plasma cells, from a case of myeloma, a malignancy of the bone marrow (see page 165).

Good examples of the essential clonality – the initiation of cancer from a single cell – do occur in human cancers. In human myeloma, a malignant bone-marrow disorder, the abnormal cells are derived from large bone marrow plasma cell clusters which normally produce two types of protein material (known as kappa and lambda), whereas in myeloma it is easy to demonstrate that either the kappa or lambda protein chain is produced, but never both (see picture, above). This points strongly towards the 'monoclonal' theory of cancer, as opposed to less dangerous types of cellular growth, for example in response to injury, in which cell regeneration is extremely important for normal recovery, but well controlled ('polyclonal' growth).

the patterns of spread in human cancer

Despite the unchecked growth so typical of cancer at the cellular level, most types of malignant or 'neoplastic' growth display some degree of predictability in their evolution and pattern of spread. In general, there are three main patterns of behaviour, with individual types of cancer tending to behave in a characteristic way, though some are more predictable than others. The major types of spread are:

- Local extension.
- Lymphatic and lymph node involvement.
- Blood-borne or 'haematogenous' dissemination.

LOCAL EXTENSION

With local invasion, a very characteristic feature of many cancers, extension takes place directly to adjacent tissue – for example, invasion of a large primary breast cancer into skin, causing ulceration, or in lung cancer, local extension to an adjacent spinal vertebra, with erosion of the bone and potential damage to the spinal cord close by. The pattern of local invasiveness may also be affected by unwise surgery. Cutting straight into a large cancer is extremely unwise and surgery of this kind is always best avoided – this is sometimes what the surgeon is rightly afraid of when he describes a cancer as inoperable, in other words, too large or attached to too many vital structures.

LYMPHATIC AND LYMPH NODE INVOLVEMENT

With lymphatic or lymph node spread, the tumour spreads initially to the local draining lymph nodes, though invasion to other nodal sites, more distant, also takes place. It is important to realise that most organs have a natural chain of draining lymph nodes, which would normally remove excess tissue fluid, deal with local infectious processes and so on. Lymph nodes in the body are often superficial, for instance in the neck or under the arm and groin. These sometimes become swollen with an infection, e.g. sore throat, but may also be affected by cancer. In cancer, invasion of local lymph nodes is common and extremely important from the point of view of prognosis. For many tumours, the presence or absence of lymph node involvement is the most important single prognostic feature, defining with considerable accuracy which patients are likely to do well and which not. In breast cancer, for example, the presence of local lymph nodes in the armpit area (the axilla, or main site of drainage of lymph nodes relating to the breast), gives valuable information to the likely outcome and helps the specialist to decide whether chemotherapy should be used. In breast cancer there is a clear, quantitative relationship between the number of lymph nodes involved and the eventual probable outcome (see page 88). In head and neck cancer, the 'lymph node status' is again a highly predictive prognostic feature and may dictate whether or not a major operation to remove these glandular areas is necessary.

HOW ELSE CAN CANCER SPREAD?

Any or all of the different patterns of spread outlined on these pages can occur together and the clinical picture then depends, of course, on the speed at which these various events take place and the precise nature of the sites involved. For instance, in patients with secondary deposits in the brain, perhaps resulting from lung, breast or large bowel cancer, the clinical picture depends critically on the specific site of the secondary, whether there is one or more, and also the rate or 'tempo' at which the dissemination has occurred. Since there are relatively 'silent' areas of the brain, i.e. areas with less critical functions than others, primary or secondary tumours can grow in these areas with much less in the way of clinical clues. For example, a tumour developing at a critical site such as the speech area, situated in the dominant hemisphere (normally the left side of the brain), would rapidly cause neurological changes.

Surgical intervention and treatment is sometimes possible with secondary brain deposits, typically where there is only one tumour visualised by scanning, and preferably in cases where it has developed at a less critical brain site, generally the lesser or non-dominant half of the brain. This is because surgical excision will be far less risky (and damaging for the patient) on the non-dominant side. In other cases (by far the majority, in fact), radiotherapy to the whole brain is a preferable form of treatment.

BLOOD-BORNE DISSEMINATION

Blood-borne or haematogenous metastasis is the most threatening type of secondary spread in cancer and is not usually curable, though there are important exceptions. Tumour deposits, possibly only single cells in the first instance, seed off from the main growth, setting down in various more or less hospitable sites within other parts of the body, and then enlarging as secondary tumours in those distant sites. Organs such as lung, bone and brain seem much more likely to harbour these deposits than, for example, heart, kidney or muscular areas of the body. Although we don't quite understand why this is, it may well be that the degree of oxygenation of the tissues at these various sites has an important bearing. What we do know, however, is that certain types of cancer have particular patterns of spread. Cancers of the head and neck areas, such as larynx, for example, tend, on the whole, to remain 'above the clavicles', so that local control of these tumours (including the important lymph node areas as well as the primary site) is usually tantamount to a cure. Breast cancer, on the other hand, has a particular predilection for spread to bone, brain, liver and lung, in addition to its local lymph node sites. Brain tumours are perhaps the most curious of all, since they may be highly malignant, with bizarre microscopic appearance and extreme difficulty in local control, particularly for the high-grade varieties, yet with almost no tendency whatsoever to metastasise to other parts of the body, and virtually no risk of lymph node invasion, even when the primary tumour cannot be surgically removed.

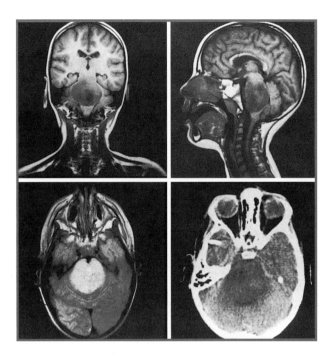

MRI scans (four views of the same patient) showing a large tumour situated at the junction of the lower part of the brain with the upper part of the spinal cord (the 'brain stem'). The remarkable detail of the normal parts of the brain is clearly displayed. For example in the bottom left scan, the tumour is visible as a large round brightly enhancing mass. Surgical removal was not possible but radiotherapy was given with good effect.

PASSAGE OF TUMOUR CELLS ACROSS A BODY CAVITY

A fourth type of spread does occasionally occur, namely passage of tumour cells across a body cavity. Although unusual in most tumours, this is an extremely important mode of spread in patients with ovarian cancer, where the predominant pattern is within the abdomen. This results from passage of tumour cells from the initial pelvic tumour upwards to the abdominal cavity itself, profoundly affecting the vital functions (such as bowel activity) within it. Despite the uncontrolled growth and abdominal distension, these patients don't usually develop secondary tumours beyond the abdominal cavity, even in the later or more extreme stages of the illness (see also pages 79–80).

In the particular group of lymphatic tumours termed 'lymphomas' (see page 149), involvement of several lymph node areas is common, whereas direct invasion and haematogenous dissemination are less important than with 'solid' malignancies, despite the frequency of bone marrow involvement in many types of lymphoma. This is also true for leukaemia, in which the dangerous consequences are largely related to 'crowding out' of the normal bone marrow elements by the malignant process itself, leading to anaemia, infection as a result of poor function or insufficient numbers of white blood cells, and a tendency towards bleeding and easy bruising, as a result of loss of platelets, those tiny marrow cells which are essential for the blood clotting process.

The partially predictable nature of cancer dissemination has led to the concept of tumour staging, which in many patients (though not all) is an important part of the initial investigation. It is important to know the true extent of any possible spread of disease before embarking on treatment, so separate tests may have to be performed to assess the extent of disease at the primary site (T), the presence of lymph node involvement (N) and also, if possible, of more distant, blood-borne metastases (M) (see box, right). For other sites, the TNM system is based on different criteria – in the breast, for instance, the T stage is deter-mined by simple measurement in centimetres of the primary tumour diameter. Brain tumours are again different, with a much greater emphasis on the grade of tumour, that is, its pathological appearance under the microscope, together with the degree to which the cells and tissue biopsy are altered from the normal appearance. In the most com-mon type of brain tumour, the group known as gliomas (see page 168), four grades are internationally recognised, with the lowest grade (grade 1) having a very good prognosis whilst grade 4 lesions are extremely difficult to treat effectively, even by surgery. It is hardly surprising that cancer specialists insist on a tissue biopsy wherever possible, in order to gain the best possible information for proper treatment.

One other important point about staging is that careful assessment of patients prior to treatment should then allow for a reasonably accu-rate comparison of results between different centres. How can you judge the claims of, say, a large American cancer centre that its new technique for brain tumours really is superior, without being sure that the patients apparently doing well are, in fact, closely comparable to those being treated at a less high-profile centre, say, in Britain or France? Although the best test of all is generally the prospectively ran-domised, controlled clinical trial, this approach is not always possible. The best we can do in such cases is to examine carefully the claims of the new treatment, to see if a large enough patient group has been treated by the new method for us to have real confidence in the results, and also to assess whether or not they were genuinely a comparable group from the point of view of tumour-related prognostic factors before the treatment was begun.

tumour staging

THE TNM STAGING SYSTEM

The TNM staging system is widely used, and specialists may speak, for example, of a T3 N1 M0 laryngeal cancer (i.e. tumour of the 'voice-box').

● T3 implies a primary tumour that is sufficiently locally advanced to have fixed the vocal cord, which is no longer as mobile as it should be.

● N1 means there is a relatively early lymph node invasion causing a palpable swelling in the neck, but not beyond a certain permissible size, which would take the stage beyond the N1 category.

● The M0 means that there is no evidence of more extensive metastatic spread.

THE PATHOLOGY OF TUMOURS

It is a common misconception that cancers are so bizarre in their appearance that the cells no longer bear any resemblance to the tissue of origin, but in fact it's the exception not the rule. For solid tumours (a curious term, but one that serves well to distinguish between the common cancers and liquid tumours, the haematological malignancies such as leukaemia), the cancer is likely to be a 'carcinoma' or, less commonly, a 'sarcoma'.

CARCINOMAS

A 'carcinoma' is a malignant tumour originating from an organ with a surface, either an external surface, such as skin, or an internal surface, such as the lining of the bronchial airways – giving rise to lung cancer – or of the lining of the upper or lower gastro-intestinal tract – resulting, for example, in a carcinoma of the stomach, oesophagus or rectum. It may seem difficult to fit breast cancer into this category, but carcinomas of the breast and other glandular organs, such as the thyroid or pancreas, are essentially carcinomas originating at the surface, or 'epithelium', of the convoluted glandular structures within. The type of carcinoma is a reflection of the initial cell of origin.

Adenocarcinomas: If the tissue of origin is obviously glandular in this way, pathologists and clinicians would regard these as adenocarcinomas. They arise from the cells of tissues in which glandular structures are a common feature.

Squamous carcinomas: The more accessible carcinomas of skin and bronchus, together with the air and food passages that make up head and neck sites, are typically squamous carcinomas. They arise from the surface or lining epithelium of cells that normally come into contact with the outside world – obvious in the case of skin, less so perhaps in the case of bronchus and rectum.

SARCOMAS

Sarcomas are primary cancer growths of soft tissue and occasionally bone, generally regarded as highly malignant in their pattern of behaviour. These tumours arise within muscle, bone or joint spaces and are difficult to characterise. Each is known separately, such as:

Leiomyosarcoma: a smooth muscle primary, such as the uterus or womb (as distinct from a uterine adenocarcinoma, much more common, where it is the lining cells of the uterus that become malignant).

Rhabdomyosarcoma: a malignant tumour of 'striped' muscle, i.e. one under voluntary active control, for instance the muscles of locomotion within the thigh or arm.

These are much less common tumours than the carcinomas, and behave in a different way. Unlike most cancers, which occur mainly in older age groups, the sarcomas that arise as primary tumours from bone sites tend to occur in adolescents. One of the greatest advances in cancer treatment during recent years is that most patients with this disorder can be treated by local surgical removal of the offending part of bone, together with chemotherapy and sometimes radiotherapy, without the need for amputation as used to be the case (see page 40).

THE CANCER CELL

The key difference between cancer and normal cells is that the normal controlling mechanisms of the cell cycle have been lost, and the cell progeny continue to grow and divide until checked by treatment – either surgical removal or an effective method of inhibiting growth, generally by radiotherapy, hormone treatment or chemotherapy. Spontaneous regressions of cancer are extremely rare. Although well documented in certain childhood tumours, a true spontaneous regression, without treatment of any kind, does not occur with a true cancer. Most cases of apparent spontaneous recovery from cancer are either treatment related or incorrectly diagnosed as cancer in the first place. As cancers become larger, they outstrip their blood supply so their innermost, least well-oxygenated cells may slow down in growth or even lose their viability altogether. Unfortunately, the rim or edge will still retain its previous capability, but there is considerable diversity in the rate of growth of tumours, some growing rather slowly, while others have a much more rapid tempo with earlier dissemination to other organs. Two major types of lung cancer illustrate this point well:

- In the typical squamous cell carcinoma, tumour growth is often relatively slow, and the specialist may for various reasons decide to watch and wait rather than immediately opt for active (and potentially hazardous) treatment in every individual case.

- On the other hand, the 'small-cell' type of lung cancer, the disease most characteristically associated with cigarette smoking, is extremely virulent and rapid in evolution, with very early dissemination to secondary sites and poor overall prognosis, despite initial responsiveness to chemotherapy.

One major cancer site, two separate types of pathology, two completely different types of malignant behaviour; and as a result, requiring quite different treatment.

TUMOUR MARKERS

Some tumours (unfortunately only a minority) produce a marker, generally a protein or other substance specific to the tumour, which is secreted into the bloodstream, and can then be detected and measured by straightforward blood tests. A good example is in testicular tumours, many of which produce two well-recognised marker substances – AFP (alpha fetoprotein) and beta HCG (human chorionic gonadotrophin) – each of which may be detectable by blood tests after apparently successful treatment of the primary tumour, even though scans may show no evidence of trouble anywhere else. In these circumstances, treatment can be given while the tumour burden is relatively modest, without waiting for other evidence of spread or recurrence of the tumour.

In other tumours we are far less fortunate, since they either fail to produce a recognisable marker or, as in the case of primary liver cancer, which may also secrete AFP, no satisfactory treatment exists, apart from surgery, for the initial primary tumour.

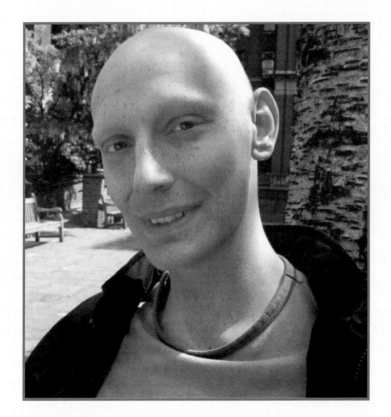

PART TWO

DIAGNOSIS AND TREATMENT

‘ *I haven't chosen this, this has chosen me, but the best thing I can do is do as much as I can to keep my life as normal as possible.* ’

GLEN XAVIER

COPING WITH THE DIAGNOSIS

symptoms

Since cancer can arise from such a wide variety of sites and develop with so many differing patterns of spread, there are no clear-cut symptoms that unequivocally give the game away. In this respect, cancer is unlike many, more specific, non-malignant ailments such as heart disease, in which chest pain, shortness of breath, exercise limitation and a few other symptoms are so often present. The arthritic diseases, characterised by joint pain and stiffness, are another good example. With cancer, the detailed symptoms depend not only on the primary site, but specifically where in the offending organ the tumour is located, the rate of development, and also whether or not secondary spread has already occurred. Occasionally, symptoms resulting from secondaries occur even before the primary site has declared itself, and amazingly enough, the initial primary from which all else has developed may sometimes never become apparent.

Many primary tumours cause local swelling if they arise at a visible or accessible part of the body, such as skin, breast, testicle or oral cavity. A tumour swelling is often painless, though ulceration (skin breakdown) can occur, which may sometimes be painful. It is important to realise that swellings in most parts of the body are generally more likely to be due to a non-malignant problem than cancer – simple viral illnesses, infectious glandular fever and so on. In the mouth, a non-healing ulcer or sore on the tongue may on the other hand mistakenly be regarded by the patient as a simple ulcer, possibly secondary to a traumatic denture, rather than being recognised as a malignant lesion.

Common symptoms and signs of cancer.

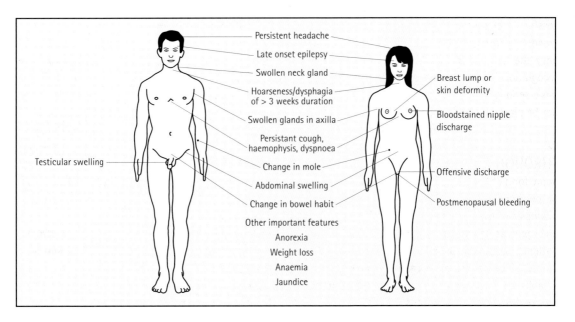

Persistent headache

Late onset epilepsy

Swollen neck gland

Hoarseness/dysphagia of > 3 weeks duration

Swollen glands in axilla

Persistant cough, haemophysis, dyspnoea

Change in mole

Abdominal swelling

Change in bowel habit

Testicular swelling

Breast lump or skin deformity

Bloodstained nipple discharge

Offensive discharge

Postmenopausal bleeding

Other important features

Anorexia

Weight loss

Anaemia

Jaundice

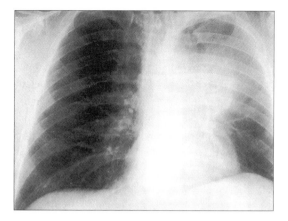

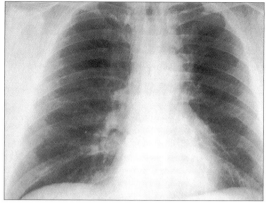

Such cases are frequently later referred on to an oral surgeon by the patient's dental practitioner.

Skin cancers produce symptoms early, unless, of course, the ulcer or swelling develops over an inaccessible site which the patient can't see – on the back or under a nail bed of one of the toes, for example. Skin tumours are dealt with in detail on pages 127-32.

With lung cancer, the symptoms may be particularly difficult to evaluate, since many smokers have chronic bronchitic complaints, with coughing, wheezing, shortness of breath and chest pain as relatively common symptoms they have become used to. It can be extremely difficult to recognise that something has genuinely changed, unless a specific complaint, such as coughing up blood, has developed, which should then alert the general practitioner to ask for a chest X-ray or a referral to a specialist. Curiously, one early feature is that patients with lung cancer often give up smoking, apparently quite easily in many cases, despite a lifetime punctuated by multiple, half-hearted or unsuccessful attempts. It happens so frequently that one can't help wondering whether there is either some innate abhorrence of cigarettes once the lung cancer has taken root or, perhaps more realistically, a recognition by the patient that this particular group of symptoms is more serious than before, even though this change in symptoms may not be picked up by the physician.

Small-cell carcinoma of the bronchus before and after treatment. This is the type of lung cancer most responsive to chemotherapy. Because it spreads early and to many parts of the body, surgical removal is very rarely recommended.

THROUGH BIOPSIES

Some form of biopsy is all-important and will almost invariably need to be performed, since it is imperative to make a firm and unequivocal diagnosis of cancer, if the patient really has it, and to then go further and gain as much information as possible. Even in elderly, infirm patients, it can be a serious mistake to treat 'on spec' without a biopsy, since sooner or later, if a watertight diagnosis hasn't been established it can become almost impossible to decide whether to proceed to additional treatment.

how is the
diagnosis made?

THE PATHOLOGIST'S REPORT

The pathologist's job is to report full technical details about the cancer, establishing the diagnosis which is essential to help direct the treatment decisions. Specialists generally regard the formal pathological diagnostic report as perhaps the most important single investigation performed during the patient's illness. The pathologist's report of cancer will be based on the appearance of the cells, their relationship to each other, the degree to which they no longer resemble cells from a normal slide of that type of tissue, and also the rate at which cells are actively dividing (the mitotic rate), which in cancer is generally higher than normal. Equally important is the observation of tumour invasiveness, with, typically, an identifiable area in which the deep layer of the tissue of origin (often termed the 'basement membrane') is clearly breached by the ingrowing tumour. This invasiveness is regarded as one of the cardinal pathological features of cancer.

The best and most secure form of biopsy is one that gives the pathologist (the specialist who peers down the microscope at microscope slide sections of tumour taken from the original block of tissue) as much material as required to make a complete diagnosis.

As a start, the patient often undergoes a simple needle biopsy as an out-patient, using local anaesthetic. Although this doesn't provide as much material as the formal histopathological specimen from a full surgical biopsy, it is usually quite sufficient to make a diagnosis of cancer with as minimal trauma to the patient as possible. In the case of skin tumours, it is often possible to remove or excise these completely, thus gaining both the diagnosis and, in many cases, adequate therapy at the same time.

In patients with lung cancer who are producing sputum from the chest, a sample of the sputum can be sent for analysis, searching for malignant cells, which might give a firm diagnosis without the need for further biopsy. In this respect, lung cancer is similar to cancer of the cervix, in which the same sort of technique, this time using a wooden spatula to gain material directly from the cervix, has been highly successful in providing a diagnosis not only of cancer, but also, in a larger proportion of cases, varying degrees of pre-cancerous change (see pages 70-1).

THROUGH FURTHER TESTS

For all the reasons discussed on pages 32-4, it is important to decide whether further information is required about the tumour before making a decision with regard to treatment. This will often involve further blood tests, X-rays, ultrasound scanning (see opposite) and/or isotope scans. What might be necessary for one type of tumour could be completely inappropriate in another; for example, in a small skin tumour of the most common types seen in the UK, no staging investigations are required at all, whereas in patients with Hodgkin's disease, one of the group of lymphomas, full scanning is required, since a patient with an enlarged gland or lymph node in the neck may have disease in the central part of the chest or even within the abdomen that is not readily visible but radiologically detectable. The most common blood tests are likely to be a full blood count, in order to check that the patient is neither anaemic nor lacking in other important blood elements, and simple blood analyses of the liver and kidney function.

THROUGH RADIOLOGY AND SCANNING

The dramatic revolution in diagnostic radiology over the past 20 years has enormously benefited cancer patients. We used to be limited to relatively simple X-rays or ultrasound scans, but now have far more sophisticated computer tomography (CT) and magnetic resonance imaging (MRI), both of which give remarkably accurate visualisation of the internal structure of various parts of the body.

CT scan: This is excellent for the chest, particularly since small secondary tumour nodules in the lungs may be seen, where a simple chest X-ray could appear normal.

MRI scan: In other parts of the body, including brain, spinal cord and pelvis, the MRI scan is likely to be superior, particularly since it can take images in virtually any plane (unlike most CT scanners) and can be repeated more frequently (since it involves no radiation exposure) to monitor progress.

Ultrasound scan: Though less glamorous perhaps than CT or MRI, ultrasound has the advantage that it is inexpensive, easy to perform, easily repeatable and without any known dangers. It is excellent for gaining information about the internal anatomy of the abdomen and pelvis, and is often used to assess whether or not the liver is involved in the cancer process. Recently, internal probes have been introduced, both for ultrasound and other types of scanning, which allow more direct and accurate inspection of the pelvis, via the oral, vaginal or rectal routes. These probes can give excellent imaging of, for example, the prostate gland sitting just beneath the bladder in men and the cervix and pelvic organs in women.

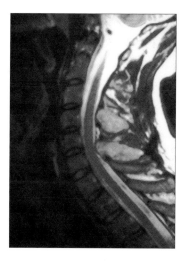

MRI scan (side view) of the upper neck showing a tumour in the spine pressing on the spinal cord, causing the clinical syndrome known as 'spinal cord compression'.

Radioactive tracers: The other important group of scanning tests involves injecting these tracers into the bloodstream (in the nuclear medicine department) followed a few hours later by scanning with a gamma-camera, which will pick up any abnormal sites or 'hot spots' (see right). This includes an exciting new form of scanner known as a PET scan (PET stands for positron emission tomography). These are just becoming more widely available and give extremely valuable information in addition to the more established methods, sometimes showing tumour activity which is otherwise undetectable.

The whole aim of this lengthy and sometimes frustrating series of investigations is to provide sufficient information for a properly informed judgement about treatment. The tests may influence the oncologist towards or away from surgery, for example, or may even point to a 'watch and wait' policy rather than immediate intervention. It is far better to take a few extra days to get this crucial information, than to rush into an inappropriate form of treatment.

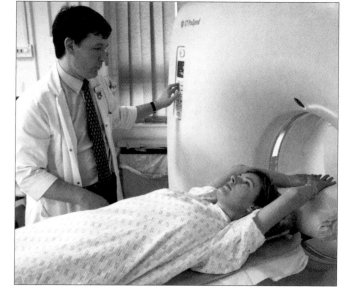

For most types of body scan the patient lies still on a couch that passes through various sensors. These produce computer-enhanced images that help the surgeon and oncologist choose the best treatment.

deciding on treatment

INITIAL DISCUSSIONS

When the treatment discussion takes place, the patient should feel free to ask any questions and should not hesitate since many specialists feel that the first one or two consultations are likely to be both the most important and, usually, the most lengthy. This may well be the best opportunity the patient has for clarification of all the issues that are bothering him or her. A good doctor should always try to avoid appearing rushed; indeed, one of the most important skills is to help the patient feel comfortable and relaxed in an extremely fraught situation and, preferably, that there is no one else in the world the doctor would sooner be with at that moment.

Patients may wish to bring a friend or family member with them for these important discussions – we don't know of any doctors who would object to this. A tape recorder can be helpful as well, though many doctors find it slightly unnerving. The only real problem with family members sitting in on the discussion is when they start to ask the questions that they want answered, without the patient voicing them him- or herself. Not a problem, perhaps, if it's a straightforward point, such as, 'How many courses of chemotherapy did you say he would probably need?', but what if the wife, sister, friend asks, 'Just how long will he have, doctor?' This isn't so easy. We're all for honesty but how does the poor doctor know whether this weighty question is one which the patient really wants to be answered?

At the end of the day, the doctor's prime responsibility is to the patient, not the family member, and if there is ever any question of conflict between them, it is the patient who is the most important person, even if, as in some cases, it is the family that is being more rational. It is the role of the companion to support, remind the patient of particular points that they had previously said they wanted to cover, perhaps to take them for a coffee afterwards, and then get them home. At a later stage it may well be necessary for both doctor and patient to repeat some of the parts of the discussion. Many other members of the multi-disciplinary team, such as nurses and therapeutic radiographers, will also be available to discuss any concerns with the patient.

In recent years, there has been an increasing acceptance of the reality and benefits of patient participation in the choice of treatment. Survival rates vary greatly from one type of cancer to another (see opposite), and have improved over the last 30 years. In certain types of cancer, cure is the rule rather than the exception though sadly, of course, these do at present remain the minority. Sharing responsibility for treatment decisions clearly has several psychological benefits for many cancer sufferers. For example, in the reduction of anxiety and depression pre- and post-operatively in patients with breast cancer, the adequacy of information supplied by the medical team seems to be the main factor in reducing both the long-term psychological consequences of the illness and the way in which it is treated.

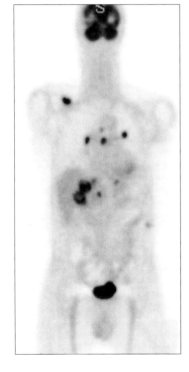

This PET scan shows tumour activity in various parts of the body including liver and lymph-node groups. The activity of the radioactive tracer in the brain and bladder is quite normal.

FOLLOW-UP DISCUSSIONS

Most cancer patients will be followed up at regular intervals after their treatment as well, gradually lessening in frequency, from diagnosis until either death or a minimum of five years. This is generally not necessary, though, for tumours that usually tend to be easily curable, such as small skin tumours.

Most patients realise that, for the first few years at least, there is often considerable uncertainty as to whether they are genuinely cured. Fortunately, most don't dwell on it; indeed, the ability to cast the uncertainty to one side is a remarkable attribute that many patients display to a most impressive degree.

One can't, of course, change one's personality, but too much broody introspection is not likely to be all that helpful, though the doctor must of course support the patient's fears and anxieties, which are likely to be expressed to their greatest degree during the first few months after treatment has been completed. Many patients, in fact, find that this is the most difficult time of all. Up to that point, they will have been 'centre stage', so to speak, and have regularly been coming to the hospital, with that powerful support of the next treatment or follow-up visit only a few weeks away. To be suddenly cast adrift at the end of it all and told that they don't need to return for two or three months can be extremely alarming, and the transformation from patient back to normality needs to be handled with great skill.

In all these discussions, both initial and follow-up, it is extremely important to avoid the use of medical jargon, a device that too many doctors hide behind. The oncology team must somehow find the right phrases, the right words, steering a path between the smoke-screen of medical terminology and unacceptable condescension.

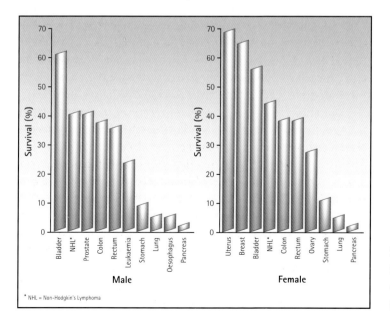

Survival (%)

Male

Female

* NHL = Non-Hodgkin's Lymphoma

Survival expectation (estimated at five years from diagnosis) in men and women with cancer, showing the great variation in outcome.

LIVING WITH UNCERTAINTY

We often read a newspaper headline 'TV soap star cured of cancer', yet halfway down the page, it becomes clear that treatment was only completed last week! Such over-simplification, to the point of trivialising the problem and insulting the readers' intelligence, does no good to any of us, least of all the TV celebrity. The truth, of course, is that years have to elapse before one can state with any certainty that a patient might genuinely be cured; the length of time depends on the nature of the cancer and the statistical probability of relapse at specific time intervals after the initial treatment.

There are some cancers that are so rapidly evolving, so lethal if untreated, that a clear passage of two years after treatment, without evidence of relapse, is all that is necessary for the patient to be declared genuinely cured. For small-cell lung cancer, for instance, and most types of testicular cancer, a clean bill of health during the two-year period, without any evidence of relapse or further medical problems, does usually mean just that. But with breast cancer, with a quite different behaviour and natural history, two years is far too short an interval; even the traditionally used five-year point is insufficient, since relapses can occur even later. Genuine advances in treatment methods will inevitably take many years of painstaking clinical research to measure and assess, and it is essential never to confuse novelty with progress.

It is uncertainty about relapse, failure of treatment and ultimately death from cancer that represent the patient's greatest fears. Repeat follow-up visits may do much to alleviate this distress, and the patient generally derives satisfaction from the knowledge that the specialist team is both competent and accessible. Many find it valuable to meet other patients who have faced the same illness, and mutual self-help groups are now very much part of the scene, some hospital based, others responding to a patient's preference to meet as far away from the hospital setting as possible.

One of the most difficult and upsetting parts of cancer medicine concerns the physical and psychological management of patients who have relapsed at a secondary site for the first time after an apparently successful initial treatment. They have moved from the position of being a potentially cured patient to one in whom cure is almost certainly no longer possible – and perhaps with a relatively limited life span. It may take far more time than is available at that single consultation, to take a view as to the best way forward and what might be the best way of imparting this knowledge to the patient, if indeed this is done at all. Although most patients will want to know the truth, there can be exceptions. Many elderly patients have no great hopes for life expectancy anyway, and have already set their affairs in order; the older generation is, perhaps, not quite as demanding of 'absolute information' at all times as those of us who are younger, more used to controlling our lives more fully, and members of different social cultures in which as much information as possible is expected. Elderly patients might be suffering from other disorders such as heart disease, which are likely to cause an earlier death than, say, a slow-growing secondary deposit from breast cancer. What is important, however, is to think carefully about the options for palliative treatment and to give the best care, regardless of whether or not it is likely to lead to a cure.

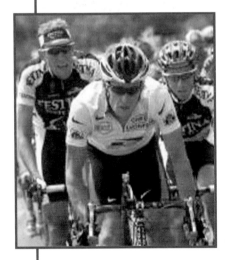

The phenomenal American cyclist, Lance Armstrong, on his way to winning the Tour de France in 1999. Only a few years before, he was diagnosed with testicular cancer, which had spread to the brain. A remarkable example of a chemotherapy cure.

HOW CAN CANCER BE TREATED?

Cancer medicine is one of the most rapidly moving of all medical specialities, both in the fields of science and understanding, and also treatment. The twentieth century saw tremendous advances in the management of cancer, particularly with the development of safer surgical techniques and the discovery, almost simultaneously, of natural radioactivity by the Curies (1898) and artificial X-ray production by Röntgen (1895). Radiation and surgery were effectively the only means of treatment during the early part of the last century, but in the 1940s, two remarkable therapeutic steps were made. First, in 1941, came the discovery of the concept of a hormone in patients with advanced prostate cancer, demonstrating for the first time that long-lasting responses could occur. And secondly, a completely new class of anti-cancer chemotherapy drugs was discovered and developed, notably nitrogen mustard, a toxic agent but with impressive activity in lymphoma and certain types of solid cancer; and a year or two later methotrexate, used from 1948 onwards for leukaemia, and producing for the first time high response rates with durable remissions in this dreaded childhood disorder.

Since that time, there has been an explosion of interest in all branches of cancer medicine, perhaps most particularly in the use of anti-cancer chemotherapy agents which, even now, are finding new applications. As little as 20 years ago, chemotherapy was still used only for a minority of cancers, whereas nowadays there are established or experimental chemotherapy protocols for virtually every type of malignant tumour. There is an important distinction between novelty and progress, yet even the natural scepticism of the British medical establishment has begun to soften. As a form of cancer treatment, chemotherapy is very much here to stay, even for selected solid tumours with only partial responsiveness.

Although many non-specialists, such as general surgeons, general physicians and gynaecologists, do see and treat cancers, with varying degrees of competence but without further referral to a specialist, there is an increasing view that patients with cancer really ought to have the opportunity of referral to a cancer specialist before firm treatment decisions are taken, even if surgical removal is the sole method of treatment required. If the surgeon initially responsible for the diagnosis and surgical treatment does not suggest referral to a specialist, ask her why. Everyone has the right to a second opinion, and who knows, it may lead to a change in policy or perhaps a more thorough assessment of the stage and other important features of the disease. Patients may have to be increasingly insistent than in the past, in order to get the advice and treatment that they have every right to expect.

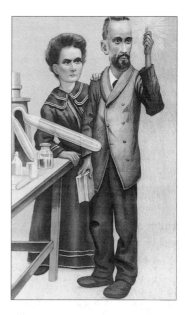

Marie and Pierre Curie with the first phial of radium, which they laboriously extracted and distilled from pitchblende. She did most of the work but he seems to be taking most of the credit!

surgery

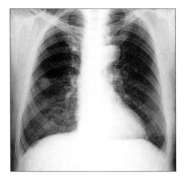

This chest X-ray shows a shadow in the mid-zone of the right lung, which proved to be an operable cancer. The surgeon was able to leave most of the lung behind, and the patient was surgically cured.

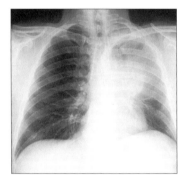

This large lung cancer was inoperable – it was too close to the main windpipe and technically could not have been removed, even if the whole of the left lung had been sacrificed.

Surgery remains an enormously important part of cancer treatment, though its role in some types of cancer has radically altered over the past 25 years. It is one of two main methods of establishing local control (the other being radiotherapy, see page 42), and the surgeon has a unique contribution to cancer management in that he or she is potentially able to completely remove or at least debulk the primary site 'at a stroke'. If cancer were always a local disease, without the problem of distant metastatic spread, the cancer surgeon would doubtless reign supreme, as in the early part of this century, when heroic surgery was frequently undertaken. Surgery is still the most effective form of treatment for certain types of cancer, notably:

● Non-small-cell lung cancer (see pages 71-3).

● Certain types of gynaecological cancer, e.g. early cancers of the cervix (see pages 80-1).

● Many skin cancers, above all melanoma (see pages 131-2).

● Most forms of soft tissue sarcoma (see pages 143-4).

● Gastro-intestinal cancers (see pages 104-7).

By and large, these are tumours in which no other method has yet proven to be superior to, or even the equal of, surgery, though in many cases – soft-tissue and bone sarcomas are good examples (see pages 143-4 and 147) – operations now are very much less radical than they used to be. Relatively conservative surgery, coupled with additional radiotherapy, chemotherapy or both, can provide as good a result in terms of survival, but with far superior functional results. Indeed, this general point holds true for much of cancer surgery today. In many areas, including genito-urinary and head and neck cancers (see pages 104-7 and 135-41), the use of early, post-operative radiotherapy has dramatically reduced the scope and extent of the surgical operation required. To give just one example, cancers of the larynx (voice apparatus) are now generally treated by radical radiotherapy (with or without chemotherapy), reserving surgery as a secondary or 'salvage' approach. The intention, of course, is to preserve the larynx and thereby the patient's normal speech function.

Perhaps the best example of the change in attitude towards surgery is in breast cancer, a disease which is unique in so many ways. Not only is it the most common of all female malignancies in the West but, most remarkably, policies for management have totally altered within the brief 25-year period from 1975. Mastectomy, so common up until that time, is now performed far more rarely, since the recognition that local tumour excision with breast preservation and early post-operative radiotherapy is at least the equal, in terms of overall survival figures, even to the most radical type of mastectomy. Second, there are now also far more effective methods of reducing the likelihood of distant relapse, using either chemotherapy or hormone approaches (see pages 47-55). Not all patients are suitable for the breast-preserving approach, but with more patients now seen with relatively small tumours (some detected by screening), patients requiring mastectomy have become the minority (see also pages 85-103).

A further important role for the surgeon lies in the second-line or 'salvage' treatment of patients where every attempt has been made to produce a cure by less drastic means, with full preservation of vital organs, but which unfortunately has been unsuccessful. Such patients aren't suitable for major surgical resection if they have already developed distant secondary spread; but relapse at the primary site, a common problem, for example, in head and neck cancers, can often be treated in this way, with as much surgical reconstruction as is feasible. Indeed, reconstructive surgery, usually a joint endeavour between oncological and plastic surgeons, has an enormous contribution to make in cancer, either as part of the initial surgical approach, or following salvage surgery of the type just mentioned.

LASER SURGERY

Laser surgery is an exciting new departure which has become frequently used in the past 15 years or so. Strictly speaking, it isn't surgery at all, at least not in the usual sense, but lasers can be used to remove blocks of tumour tissue, and are quite often used in accessible head and neck cancers, such as the tongue, as well as in removal of areas of early cervical cancer or pre-cancer. Major advances have been made with laser treatment of lung and gullet (oesophageal) cancers, since conventional surgical treatment may be unsuitable and the laser is capable of burning through completely blocked areas, then allowing local radiotherapy an opportunity for more long-term control. In cancer of the oesophagus, for example, patients quite often have such severe blockage that they may have lost more than 10% of their body weight and be unable to swallow any food at all. This dire situation can be rapidly reversed by laser application (easily repeatable if necessary), with re-establishment of the channel, relief of the blockage, and early treatment with radiotherapy.

The consequences of surgery for specific sites (for example, the management of the patient after mastectomy and availability of prostheses and reconstructive services) are dealt with in the specific chapters.

POST-TREATMENT CONSEQUENCES

Following surgical operations for cancer, the recovery period is usually fairly rapid, depending, of course, on the site, extent and scope of the surgery. Many patients are out of hospital within a week or so following standard procedures such as mastectomy, hysterectomy or exploratory abdominal operations. Other operations may take a bit longer – removal of a lung or a bowel resection, for instance. Major and complicated operations, particularly those in the head and neck region that require surgical reconstruction, are inevitably more taxing and generally require a longer period both in hospital and for recovery.

Complex procedures are generally best undertaken at special centres where the appropriate teams of surgeons, working in co-operation, are available – and well used to working with each other.

Always ask your surgeon about the likely consequences of an operation and how long it will take for recovery. It might also be a good opportunity to let the surgeon know that whatever the outcome, you would like to hear the results of the operation and to know about what the pathologist found when he or she examined the specimen. You may not wish to do this, of course, and many patients feel inhibited from asking these questions, since they feel 'it's not their place' even though they would like to have the information. This simply won't do! You have to be bolder than that if you want to participate in your care and be kept well informed. You may not wish to – and, of course, you don't have to – but there is no need to feel that information about your own body, your own state of health, is somehow not your business. You may wish to take a relative or friend along to the consultation or have the opportunity to speak to a specialist nurse after the consultation or on the reception.

radiotherapy

Although a more recent speciality than surgery, with a history stretching back only 100 years, radiotherapy has become the pre-eminent form of treatment for many of the common cancers, and is now used for more than 50% of patients, this number steadily rising. Remarkably, the first attempt at using radiotherapy for skin and other cancers came within a few weeks of its discovery, and by 1924, the great British surgeon Sir Geoffrey Keynes had already started examining its potential in breast cancer – happily he lived on to the age of 94, quite long enough to see it established and also his prediction of the decline of mastectomy fulfilled. Improvements in radiotherapy equipment, technique and applications have led to an increasing role both in local treatment (in many cases, supplanting surgery or reducing the need for radical operations) and also in its use as a whole-body treatment, as part of bone marrow transplantation techniques for leukaemia and other malignant diseases (see page 57).

The radiotherapist has to try to achieve the best possible compromise between damaging the cancer cell and the normal surrounding host tissues – never an easy task since a high dose, often very close to the tolerance of normal organs, may be necessary to achieve a cure, particularly with the common solid tumours treated every day. Good examples of cancers successfully treated by radiotherapy are:

- Cervical cancer (see page 83).
- Bladder cancer (see pages 118-19).
- Prostate cancer (see pages 121-2).

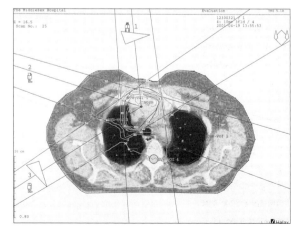

A typical example of a modern radiotherapy plan, showing the disposition of the radiotherapy beams displayed on a CT-scan 'slice' of the patient at mid-chest level, and the radiation dose within the relevant normal tissues as well as the tumour itself.

HOW DOES RADIOTHERAPY WORK?

X-rays and gamma rays lie at the most energetic end of the electro-magnetic spectrum, with a short wavelength and a high energy. Unlike all other energy waves, such as visible light, ultraviolet or radio waves, X-rays have sufficient energy to cause profound disruption of mammalian (including human) tissue cells. Although this applies not only to tumour cells but also normal tissues, there is a real and exploitable difference between the limited capability of the tumour to withstand the X-ray assault and recover from it, and the much greater healing properties of normal tissues. Whether this difference results chiefly from an intrinsically greater radiation sensitivity for tumour tissue, or a better power of recovery for normal cells, remains somewhat in doubt. The net result, however, is that X-ray treatment of many cancers, when properly carried out with great attention to detail of target volume and dose, can often sterilise tumour tissue while producing a completely acceptable degree of side-effects. A good example is in early cancer of the larynx (and fortunately the majority of cases of laryngeal cancer in the Western world fall into this category), a tumour in which radiation cure is achievable in over 90% of cases, without any loss of function or serious injury to the voice. This figure is closely comparable with the degree of cure from surgery, but radiotherapy is obviously preferable whenever possible, because of its greater degree of patient acceptability. Surgery is generally reserved (in the UK at least) for radiation failure.

- Breast cancer (see pages 90-3).
- Some types of lung cancer (see pages 71-4).

EXTERNAL RADIATION THERAPY

Over the past decade or so, tremendous advances in imaging techniques, notably with computer tomography (CT) and magnetic resonance imaging (MRI), have permitted treatments to become much more precise. For instance, before CT scanning, patients with a malignant brain tumour generally required very wide field radiation therapy, to be sure of covering the whole area adequately. Nowadays, with much improved tumour localisation, the normal surrounding tissues can be avoided more effectively, concentrating a higher dose more safely on the smaller volume that needs to be treated.

To complement improvements in tumour localisation, advances in radiotherapy equipment have allowed radiation to be delivered to virtually any site in the body, with a much lower dose to the surrounding sensitive tissues. The skin can usually be avoided – an important point, since it was the skin burning that so limited the radiation dose during the early part of the last century.

INTERNAL RADIATION THERAPY

Internal radiation therapy can be delivered by mouth, passed into a body orifice (or through the skin) or, in some cases, by using a radiation implant actually passed into the tumour itself. This is known as brachytherapy. In cancer of the thyroid, for example, the fact that the thyroid gland is the only part of the body which will take up iodine (and therefore radioactive iodine as well) can be exploited by deliberately giving radioactive iodine by mouth. It will immediately home in on the thyroid gland in the neck and cause the gland and its cancer to 'self-destruct'. A true 'magic bullet' indeed!

COMBINED TREATMENTS

Radiation can be used with other types of cancer treatment as well, in combination with surgery and laser therapy (see page 41), chemotherapy (see overleaf) or hormones (see page 54). Some cancers are routinely treated by a combination of external beam and implant therapy, the implant being used to boost the tumour dose to a higher level at the primary site. As ever, the trick is to achieve maximum tumour cell destruction with minimal side-effects to normal tissues.

In breast cancer: Radiation is given to patients who have undergone local excision and breast preservation since local excision surgery alone is less adequate in terms of local control of disease than what was previously achieved by mastectomy (see page 90).

In childhood tumours: There are some tumours in which radiotherapy was previously regarded as essential, but can now be safely avoided. Radiotherapy can be hazardous in childhood tumours because of growth retardation; most solid childhood cancers other than brain tumours are responsive to chemotherapy (chemosensitive) and radiotherapy is now used far less frequently in children, for example in those with non-Hodgkin's lymphoma and Wilms' tumour (see pages 153-8 and 187-8). However, the increased use of brain (cranial) irradiation or, in some cases, treatment of both the brain and spinal cord has dramatically improved the overall cure rate for childhood brain tumours.

In bone marrow transplantation: Radiotherapy is increasingly being used as a 'systemic' form of treatment, notably in combination with bone marrow transplantation – the idea here being that for patients with a poor outlook from certain types of leukaemia, multiple myeloma and lymphoma it may be possible to perform a bone marrow transplant. The patient's own bone marrow, or marrow from a closely matched donor (preferably a twin, if one is available – see John's story on page 56) is removed and stored, then the patient is treated with either chemotherapy, radiotherapy, or both, in high doses. The marrow is then returned, repopulating the marrow space within the body and re-forming the essential bone marrow elements over the next few weeks. If it is necessary to use donated bone marrow from a relative, this will ensure that the marrow will not be contaminated by residual tumour, but it's much more difficult in practice, because of the need to suppress immunity (since the graft is 'foreign' tissue) during the post-transplant period (see also page 57).

Although it is the bone marrow transplant that is the 'glamorous' part of such treatments, it is, of course, the high doses of total body irradiation and chemotherapy that provide the real cure – the transplant simply provides the technological means of keeping the patient alive, or so it is believed. More recently, it looks as though it might be possible to do away with marrow transplants altogether, by using circulating blood cells stimulated by certain biological growth factors in order to bring out the powerful 'precursor' cells from the marrow into the bloodstream – already a reality in some cancers.

In palliative treatment: For patients with widespread disease in whom cure is unrealistic, palliative radiotherapy is generally the most valuable of treatments available and is used in a wide variety of clinical settings, particularly for painful or unstable bone deposits. It is often used together with orthopaedic internal fixation, a highly effective combination providing both mobility and freedom from pain.

THE SIDE-EFFECTS OF RADIOTHERAPY

Although the ability to deliver effective radiotherapy without serious side-effects has clearly been improved, there is still a long way to go. Too often, a radiation cure has its price in terms of both short and long-term toxicity. In the short term, acute effects, such as diarrhoea, skin discomfort and abdominal cramping from pelvic irradiation, should be relatively easy to deal with, particularly if short lived. It is the longer term side-effects that are more disturbing. For some patients (fortunately the minority), the price of a radiation cure for an otherwise lethal pelvic cancer (cervix, bladder and so on) can include long-term bowel damage, occasionally leading to such severe radiation consequences that the affected part of the bowel has to be removed, and the patient provided with a colostomy. Sadly, it is impossible to ensure that cure can be achieved without damage of this kind occurring from time to time – a consequence of biological variability within different patients. However, lowering the dose to a level that would never produce damage would reduce radiation cure rates to an unacceptably low level as well.

When it comes to more specific cancer treatments, such as radiation and chemotherapy, patients are generally warned in advance that they might suffer certain consequences (for chemotherapy side-effects, see page 48). How far should the specialist go in warning patients of potential undesirable consequences? If, for example, a radiation side-effect is universal, such as hair loss following irradiation for a brain tumour, it would be wrong and unfair to fail to warn the patient, though advising how long it might take before re-growth occurs is always a problem, since it can be so variable. If, on the other hand, a complication is extremely unusual, but very occasionally occurs, should one frighten every patient by pointing out that it could happen? A good example of this would be the radiation damage, particularly the arm weakness, that can occur as a result of irradiation of nervous tissue during radiotherapy treatment for breast cancer. Only a tiny minority of women have suffered this side-effect, though on occasion it has produced devastating consequences. Should all patients be warned about this? Would it do more good than harm? Might they unwisely forgo a critically important part of their treatment because of an unreasonable fear? These are not easy questions, particularly since many radiotherapists will never have seen a single case in their own personal practice, even with many years' experience.

Perhaps the patient should decide, when meeting the radiotherapist for the first time, just how much he or she wishes to know about the potential dangers, as well as the possible benefits. Obviously no one should treat any patient unless the benefits are likely to outweigh the disadvantages, but the patient may well need reassurance. It is extremely unfortunate to cure a patient of cancer and yet face their anger and dismay if a serious radiation side-effect has developed, which they feel they weren't adequately warned about.

POST-TREATMENT CONSEQUENCES

Serious radiation damage is fortunately unusual, though the need to keep dosage high for best tumour effect does, of course, mean that moderate side-effects are often encountered.

Cancer in the head and neck: In irradiating tumours here, for example, large volumes of the lining of the mouth and/or throat may have to be treated, with irritation, soreness and dryness of these surfaces commonly occurring as an acute reaction. During treatment it might be difficult to swallow, so liquid diets, nutritional support from a specialist dietician, and even nasogastric tube feeding or a specially positioned stomach tube may be necessary. This type of support can make all the difference to successful treatment without severe weight loss. These methods of support are often essential since, for a patient with locally advanced cancer in the head and neck region, there is still a chance of cure, even without surgery, provided that the radiation (and, in some instances, chemotherapy) is given to a sufficiently intensive dose. As so often, it is the supportive care that makes possible the full delivery of the scheduled anti-cancer treatment.

In lung cancer: Radiation therapy for lung cancer may also cause difficulties with swallowing, because of the direct radiation effect on the oesophagus. It is usually possible to help with antacids and other medicines, which line the oesophagus and give a soothing local anaesthetic effect. Oncology departments run a strict policy of assessing each patient regularly throughout treatment – this is your opportunity to let the specialist or those treating you such as the nurse or radiographer know whether symptoms are developing, so that they can be urgently treated.

In liver, small bowel, stomach and kidney cancers: In the abdomen, the limited radiation tolerance of many of the organs has led to a particularly cautious use of radiotherapy. The abdomen chiefly remains the province of the surgeon when it comes to primary treatment, though many tumours spread within this part of the body and secondary treatments, generally with some form of chemotherapy, are commonly attempted.

In the pelvis: Here radiation has an extremely important role both in gynaecological tumours (particularly cervix and uterus) and for 'genitourinary' sites, such as bladder and prostate. Because of the limited radiation tolerance of the lower bowel (rectum) and other structures close by, this is an exceptionally difficult site to treat without complications. The patient's life is all too often genuinely at stake, since treatment by radiotherapy may represent the only possible chance of cure as so many patients unfortunately have inoperable disease. Undesirable consequences of radiation do occur from time to time, even in the best hands – unless, of course, the therapist is prepared to lower the radiation dose and accept more treatment failures as the price of never causing this type of damage.

chemotherapy

In many ways, the twin developments of chemotherapy and hormone therapy (see page 54) represent the most exciting advances of all over the past 40 years. Before the mid-1950s, patients with disseminated cancer, leukaemia or lymphoma invariably died of it. By contrast, substantial groups of patients are regularly expected to be cured, including those with Hodgkin's disease, many of the non-Hodgkin's lymphomas, leukaemias and childhood cancers, and the overwhelming majority of patients with testicular tumours. Celebrated sportsmen with disseminated cancer have won the Grand National and the Tour de France, possibly the most gruelling sports event in the world. Even where cure is still not possible, the advent of chemotherapy has often provided an improvement in survival and lengthy remission. This group includes:
- Ovarian cancer (see pages 80-3).
- Myeloma (see page 166).
- Some of the non-curable lymphomas (see pages 155-6).
- Many types of lung cancer (see pages 71-4).
- Breast cancer (see pages 95-6).

Most exciting of all, perhaps, is the demonstration that in tumours like breast cancer, which are only moderately responsive to chemotherapy, its early use (as 'adjuvant' therapy given directly after surgery) does clearly improve the outlook, with a statistically watertight improvement in survival documented as far out as 15 years from diagnosis and initial treatment, even though the adjuvant chemotherapy had generally been given for a total of only six months at the start of the illness. This observation was the product of lengthy and painstaking international co-operation and speaks volumes for the enormous power of well-conducted clinical trials. This has given the lead in many other cancer areas, where specialists are trying to replicate this advantage by testing chemotherapy in other settings. Colorectal cancer, for example, is of considerable current interest because, like breast cancer, it has a relatively marginal response to chemotherapy; yet its early use, when the tumour burden is at its minimum following surgery, seems again to be working, though its track record so far is nowhere near as well documented as that of breast cancer.

Cancer treatment with effective cell-killing ('cytotoxic') therapy has much to contribute, yet the word 'chemotherapy' strikes dread into the hearts of many patients. It still seems to have a bad press for two reasons. First, it was used far too indiscriminately in the early days, in the vain hope that it could cure every malignant ailment, however advanced. Hopefully, treatment has moved on from the indiscriminate and largely valueless use of chemotherapy in situations where there could be no justification other than the physician's desire to 'do something'. Second, it is still widely perceived (wrongly!) that all patients receiving chemotherapy inevitably suffer the most terrible consequences from side-effects.

THE SIDE-EFFECTS OF CHEMOTHERAPY

In truth, the side-effects of chemotherapy are much misunderstood, so here is an outline of the main side-effects.

Nausea and vomiting: Only a small proportion of chemotherapy drugs cause really severe nausea and vomiting, and the good news is that, during the 1990s, a new class of more effective anti-nausea preparations, which work by antagonising the trigger chemical causing nausea, have become widely available. Since most forms of chemotherapy act to some extent as cell poisons, it is perhaps not surprising that nausea and vomiting are such frequent symptoms. Several chemo drugs can cause this distressing side-effect, with three in particular, doxorubicin, cisplatin and nitrogen mustard (mustine) among the worst offenders. Most of the drugs that can be given by mouth, such as cyclophosphamide, busulphan, melphalan and methotrexate, are much less troublesome. In truth, however, the reason for chemotherapy-induced emesis isn't very well understood, though there appears to be a centrally located area in the brain triggered off by the stimulus of chemotherapy. However, even powerful intravenous drugs, which can cause serious nausea and vomiting, are generally tamed by the new supportive anti-emetic agents (see pages 53 and 207).

Hair loss: The second most feared side-effect is hair loss, which again is a feature of only a rather small proportion of chemotherapy drugs in

CHEMOTHERAPY DRUGS

For the most part, these drugs fall into specific categories, with mechanisms of action which, in many cases, are reasonably well understood. Some act by inhibiting the DNA cleavage that precedes tumour cell division; they do this by tight binding of the DNA components, preventing the chromosomal material within the tumour cell from being properly incorporated into the next generation of cells. Many of these drugs have been in common use for 30 years and few have severe side-effects (see below) if taken at the correct dose. Other chemo drugs are simple analogues or 'look-alikes' of biological base materials that would normally be incorporated into the DNA of an active tumour cell. These drugs, often termed 'anti-metabolites', seem to work by being incorporated into the tumour cell directly; when cell division is attempted, the true nature of the cellular antagonist or 'look-alike' drug is revealed, and the DNA division is halted.

Combinations of drugs generally work better, presumably by providing an opportunity to block the metabolic pathway of the cancer cell more effectively, at a number of separate biochemical stages. Chemotherapy schedules (or 'protocols') employ agents from different categories in order to gain the maximum cell kill with a minimum of side-effects.

common use. It is regrettable, of course, but excellent wigs are now available, hair loss (alopecia) is often only partial, and the best news of all is that the alopecia caused by cancer chemotherapy is invariably temporary. The hair always comes back, one of the few absolute guarantees that the oncologist can give, and when it grows back it's often wavier or curlier than before. For more information, see page 201.

Bone marrow suppression: This is common with cancer chemotherapy, but generally not to the point of danger. Again, advances in supportive care have greatly helped to tide patients over a temporary period of bone marrow failure. As the marrow produces blood cells, the effects include:
- Anaemia, which can be relieved by blood transfusion if required.
- Lowering of the white cell count (the anti-infection defence cells), which can be countered by antibiotics and, if necessary, biological growth factors.
- A bleeding tendency from loss of the platelet cells of the blood, usually dealt with, if necessary, by platelet transfusions, which can be given until the danger period is passed.

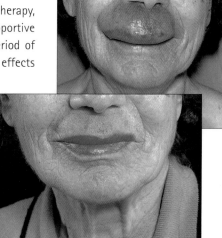

Other side-effects: Other types of chemotherapy agent have specific side-effects not shared by all of the drugs. For example, several of the drugs can cause troublesome but reversible pins-and-needles by affecting the nerves in the hands and feet, while cisplatin, a chemically simple heavy-metal complex that has transformed many types of cancer, can damage the kidney and cause deafness. Oncology specialists have learnt how to use these agents more safely, however –

In this case of NHL (non-Hodgkin's lymphoma) of the upper lip, chemotherapy produced a dramatic response within a few weeks. Rather to our surprise, further treatment with radiotherapy proved unnecessary.

SAM'S STORY

Sam is a 20-year-old student from north London. In his gap year, he went to Africa where he took part in a teaching project. It was during the last two weeks of the trip, while he was enjoying some time out travelling around with his friends, that he awoke one morning and noticed that his elbow was extremely painful.

When Sam returned to Britain he went to his GP who diagnosed tendonitis. The pain did not disappear, however, and he was then referred to the physiotherapist in case he had a trapped nerve. He had two weeks of intensive physiotherapy. By now Sam found it difficult to grip a pen and to cut up his food and he found that he could not straighten his arm either. Despite this, Sam went on to start his philosophy course at university but one night he went to the Accident and Emergency department at the hospital because he was in so

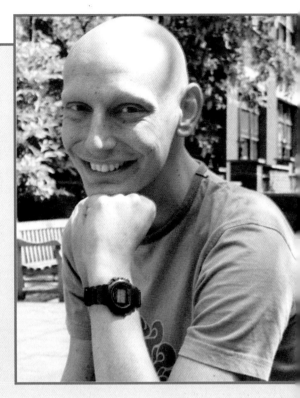

much pain. An X-ray was performed, but did not show anything. On Halloween night, Sam went out with some friends to a club and had a few drinks and the next morning he awoke to find himself in hospital having fallen over and fractured his affected arm. An MRI scan was performed and later on that day he was told that the scan had shown that it could well be a cancerous tumour in his arm.

Sam had suspected something was wrong but never that it might be cancer. He recalls that he felt relieved that they had put a name to what was wrong. 'I just thought, people get tumours all the time and they are not usually malignant. I sort of thought, well, gosh, damn, it might be cancer but it probably won't be. It slowly crept over me that actually it was verging on the probable that it was cancer. They did a biopsy, which diagnosed the tumour to be a Ewing's sarcoma and by then I'd sort of gone into the state of mind where I was pretty resigned to it. When I did know it was cancer it was like, well, I'll take a year off and then start again. So I thought that's OK. This is all an experience, what an experience. I'm, like, 19 years old and I've got cancer. But I wasn't devastated.'

Sam felt that his family were more upset at the diagnosis than he was. He felt, 'It's me, it's happening to me and if I'm not upset, it was almost as if nobody else had the right to be upset and I realised afterwards, of course, they have got a right to be upset. I was like just accepting and ready to start the battle.' When he told his old friends and the many new friends from his year in Africa that he had cancer he found by and large that they were shocked and at first didn't know what to do or say, but given time Sam has found that they and his family have been very supportive. Sam says that it's a funny part of being seriously ill that you have to be reassuring and calm others down. He finds it refreshing when people are just up front and say, 'My God Sam, I heard you've got cancer. How did that happen?' and just have a normal and open conversation about it.

Sam decided to leave university and return home to London for treatment for the cancer. He underwent further investigations prior to starting the chemotherapy, which detected metastatic disease in the lung and an abnormality in the bone of the sacro-iliac joint. Sam subsequently underwent chemotherapy on the

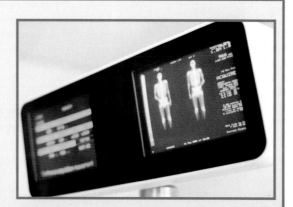

Teenage Cancer Trust Unit and although he was prepared for the side-effects of the treatment he was troubled by nausea and became confused and hallucinated during the first treatment. He then became neutropenic and developed an infection so he ended up in hospital for nearly three weeks. Sam also lost his hair during the treatment. 'It's quite funny to lose all your bodily hair, but it doesn't bother me at all. It's not so nice in winter because it's so cold, but in the warmer months it's really nice.' The medical staff decided it would be worthwhile reducing the dose of the chemotherapy for the subsequent cycles so although he still suffered side-effects they were not so severe as they were before.

After the sixth cycle of chemotherapy, an operation was planned to remove the tumour in Sam's arm. Unfortunately, the scan showed that the tumour was not responding to the chemotherapy as it had before, so the operation was postponed and Sam was given a further two courses of another combination of chemotherapy.

Sam has now undergone surgery to his arm and will be having high dose chemotherapy and a peripheral blood stem cell transplant, which will require him to stay in hospital for about three weeks. He is, however, looking forward to completing his treatment so that if all goes to plan he can then start his philosophy degree again in a few months, but this time at Edinburgh University.

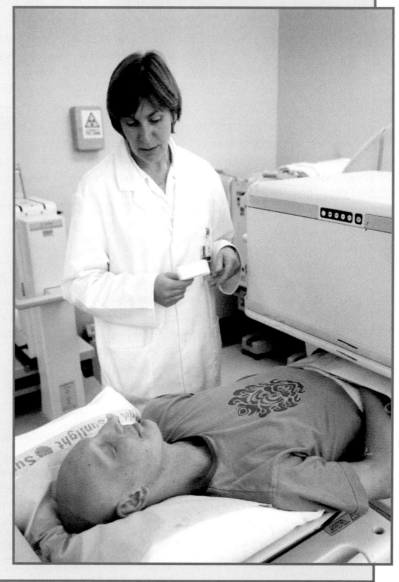

in the case of cisplatin, for example, by providing adequate hydration with intravenous fluids whenever it is used, and, if really necessary, by use of an alternative cisplatin derivative drug (carboplatin), which has fewer of these side-effects. Specialists in drug development both in university settings, hospitals and the pharmaceutical industry, have been extremely ingenious in recognising the limitations of current cancer chemotherapy and finding ways to overcome them.

THE LONG-TERM CONSEQUENCES

Long-term consequences of chemotherapy can be important and so it is imperative the patient understands what might happen. When faced with the offer of chemotherapy for the first time, it is reasonable for the patient to ask, 'How much benefit and at what personal cost?' Specialists are there to answer questions just as much as to dish out the treatment, and should be happy to engage in a two-way dialogue. In any event, even if they aren't keen, you, the patient, have a right to know. As so often in this book, the advice is: 'If you have a question, then don't hesitate to ask.'

Infertility: A number of the chemotherapy agents can cause infertility – not a problem for the majority of cancer patients, who are likely to be over 40 years of age, but certainly a major issue in younger ones, whose prospect for cure may depend entirely on the effectiveness of chemotherapy if the disease is too widespread to be curable by local irradiation. Men, in particular, seem to be affected in this respect, since spermatic precursors (the cells from which mature sperm cells are derived) seem to be relatively easily damaged. Any young man faced with cancer chemotherapy for, say, Hodgkin's disease or other conditions should be warned about this and have the opportunity for sperm storage – an easy technological task, though some patients, particularly those with testicular tumours, have a low sperm count, which makes sperm banking impossible.

SARAH'S STORY

Sarah was 28 when she first went to her doctor for a smear test and naturally became concerned when she was recalled. Clearly, the test hadn't been normal, but initially it looked as though there was no great cause for alarm. It seemed sensible, though, to arrange for a colposcopy, and the gynaecologist was indeed surprised to find a visible abnormality which, of course, he biopsied. This turned out to show the highest grade of cervical pre-cancer (CIN 3), so he arranged for a cone biopsy. Sadly, the biopsy showed not a pre-cancerous, but a true micro-invasive cancer, for which radical hysterectomy would certainly be the correct form of treatment.

Sarah was devastated. It was as if, at each stage, the reassurances she had previously been given proved utterly false; her thoughts, dreams and prayers for motherhood had turned to dust. Worse was to come. At what should have been a curative operation, enlarged glands were noted in the pelvic side wall, subsequently proving, after a biopsy, to harbour unexpected metastatic lymph node deposits.

Her oncology specialist had to break the news and explain the need for further treatment, which he felt should consist of both abdomino-pelvic irradiation and chemotherapy. They had a long, painful discussion, with tears and many questions from Sarah. 'Will chemotherapy make my hair fall out? Will the radiotherapy dry up my ovaries? Will I be infertile? Could this cancer kill me?' Yes, yes, yes and yes. You could hardly describe Sarah as lucky, but she did at least have a tremendously supportive husband and good friends. After the initial discussion with her specialist, and a couple more like it to go through the details once again, Sarah stuck out her jaw and then her forearm (for the drip) and told him to get on with it.

Ten years on, Sarah is cured. She and her husband have moved house (they now live in the country) and have adopted two daughters.

For women, the risk of infertility seems to be lower. But with the increasing use of adjuvant chemotherapy for breast cancer, this has become a major issue for women of child-bearing age. Patients should know that the chemotherapy might disturb the periods and could interrupt them altogether, without the certainty of spontaneous recovery. In general, though, the younger the woman, the less likely she is to be rendered completely infertile. It is now becoming possible to store unfertilised eggs, as with the easy storage of sperm.

Kidney damage: Other long-term consequences of chemotherapy include permanent renal (kidney) damage, nowadays less of a problem since the main offending drug, cisplatin, is better understood and used more safely with adequate fluid hydration.

Lung damage: This can occur when the drug bleomycin is used. It is a widely used agent for testicular, head and neck and some of the pelvic and lung cancers.

POST-TREATMENT CONSEQUENCES
Although chemotherapy has traditionally had a bad press from the point of view of side-effects, enormous improvements have been made over the past ten years.

Overcoming nausea and vomiting: The treatment of chemotherapy-induced emesis (nausea and vomiting) and of the bone marrow consequences (leading to dangerous reduction of the circulating blood elements) is now much more effective. With the anti-nausea drug domperidone available, most patients are well enough to cope pretty well, without needing in-patient care, often getting back to work within a day or two of the chemotherapy.

Helping bone marrow suppression: Bone marrow suppression is, if anything, a more serious problem, less upsetting for the patient perhaps, but potentially far more dangerous. Most of the chemotherapy drugs do cause a degree of temporary bone marrow failure, fortunately short-lived in most cases. However, just as radiation oncologists are rightly obsessed by delivering the proper dose for the best possible effect, specialists in cancer chemotherapy generally prefer to give high doses since this is likely to lead to a much-improved response. The traditional barrier to such high-dose treatment has been the inability of the bone marrow to cope, leading to dangerous periods of suppression of the white cells, which are essential for defence against infection (neutropenia) and also a reduction in the platelet count, leading to bruising and bleeding. Anaemia also occurs, but is easily reversible by blood transfusion. In patients with fragile bone marrow reserve, such as those with acute leukaemia, it is extremely important to treat with antibiotics, generally by intravenous administration, if the patient becomes neutropenic and develops a fever, even before the infectious cause has been established, since there is simply no time to lose.

In patients with solid tumours, whose bone marrow reserve is normal, one can usually be a little more relaxed, assuming of course that conventional doses of anticancer chemotherapy have been given and that early bone marrow recovery can confidently be predicted. The ability to deliver higher doses safely has been greatly advanced by the development of biological substances, generally known as cytokines, which are mostly bone marrow stimulators of various types. These agents enhance bodily defences, assisting the natural substances that are responsible for bone marrow recovery. Most of these 'biological response modifiers' work on the white cell series and are generically known as colony stimulating factors (CSFs). Attempts to improve the early recovery of platelets have been less successful, however, though platelet transfusions are freely available and are capable of tiding patients over brief periods (i.e. timespans of less than a month) of severe platelet suppression.

hormone therapy

With hormone therapy, the situation is altogether different to that of chemotherapy. Less widely used than chemotherapy, it is often seen as the 'gentler alternative'. The truth is that its indications are much more limited, since only a small minority of tumours are hormone sensitive and these include breast cancer (see pages 93-5) and prostate cancer (see page 121).

As with chemotherapy, only a proportion of patients respond, and it is generally impossible to determine in advance which these might be, with the exception of breast cancer, where it is possible to use the reasonably reliable oestrogen receptor assay technique, performed quite simply on the original biopsy in the pathology department. The great advantage of hormone therapy is that it provides a systemic means of treatment, i.e. to the whole body, but without the side-effects of chemotherapy. Furthermore, hormone-induced responses are often remarkably durable, often more so than with chemotherapy. For example, in breast cancer, a highly hormone-sensitive patient with metastatic or secondary disease may enjoy years of good-quality life as a result of control of the secondary tumours by hormone manipulation, whereas chemotherapy in such circumstances tends to have a more short-lived effect. For this reason, even though response rates to hormone therapy in breast cancer are lower than with chemotherapy, hormone therapy nonetheless tends to be preferred, wherever possible – though sometimes, as pointed out above, it simply isn't logical.

The anti-oestrogen tamoxifen, which is extremely active and is given by mouth to the majority of patients with breast cancer, has very few side-effects, and has been an established part of treatment for over

QUALITY OF LIFE ISSUES IN CANCER

No one would dispute the fact that, to achieve a cure from cancer, most patients would be prepared to put up with almost any degree of treatment-related side-effects, provided they came through in the end. While it is certainly justifiable to put patients through a very tough time if there is simply no alternative to achieve a cure, what about patients for whom cure is only a remote possibility? How do we help yet make sure that in our enthusiasm to do what we can, we don't do more harm than good?

Oncologists have long been aware of this dilemma; indeed, some of the earliest studies in Hodgkin's disease, dating from the 1960s, recognised the extremely nauseating effects of the relatively primitive (but sometimes effective) chemotherapy, and attempted to substitute effective, but less nauseating, drugs for the worst offenders. This has led to newer and more acceptable regimens for Hodgkin's disease, which are substantially still in use today. Although the newer treatment is no better in terms of effectiveness, it is certainly far less nauseating and therefore much more acceptable to patients. More recently, those working in the quality-of-life area have attempted to define methods of measuring this elusive component of our daily lives (everyone knows what it means but few can put it exactly into words!). Generally, these assessments depend on patient questionnaires, but there are also methods by which patients enter a mark on a simple linear analogue scale ('How well do you feel today, on an arbitrary scale of 1 to 10?'). This technique can be expanded to cover many specific questions concerning mood, physical comfort, freedom from specific complaints such as nausea, breathlessness, constipation and so on, and many other areas.

The whole topic is brilliantly dealt with in Professor Lesley Fallowfield's book *The Quality of Life* (Souvenir Press, 1990), which both addresses the general issues of the quality of life and also takes doctors to task for quite frequently disregarding it. It is certainly important to recognise at all times whether one's enthusiastic use of dangerous and discomforting drugs is always justified, particularly in diseases like extensive small-cell lung cancer (see page 73) where cure is only a remote possibility. It is even more important to recognise that the patient's quality of life, given that the total time is likely to be limited, is of much greater importance perhaps than a few extra weeks of life. Needless to say, patients do vary considerably in their views on this matter, and some prefer every attempt to be made regardless of personal cost, particularly if they wish – as so often seems the case – to witness a particular event such as the birth of a grandchild, a daughter's wedding and so on. Many patients are quite frank about these matters, and rightly expect a corresponding degree of candour on the part of the physician treating them. Most patients much prefer honesty, even if the news is disappointing, to evasiveness or an elaborate discussion cloaked with half truths. It is all to the good that, during the past decade, there has been increasing attention to the quality of life in patients undergoing cancer treatment. For many patients, quality of life is highly dependent on their physical condition, and every attempt must be made to reduce the negative and highly debilitating side-effects of cancer and its treatment.

a decade, at least in post-menopausal patients. It has considerably improved survival and reduces the risk of a 'contralateral' primary, i.e. development of a new breast cancer on the other side. As it is so active and relatively free of side-effects, it is now being used as a means of attempting prevention of breast cancer development in those regarded as being at high risk (usually by virtue of a very strong family history in an otherwise normal subject) – quite properly, within a randomised controlled trial setting (see also page 210).

JOHN'S STORY

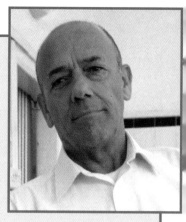

John is a 63-year-old butcher, who lives with his wife in Potter's Bar. He had always been fit and enjoyed good health but for a while he had been seeing his GP about a minor but irritating ailment that was being treated with various anti-inflammatory tablets. At one of their regular consultations, the GP decided that John should have a routine blood test. The very same day John was informed that the results of the test showed he needed to be admitted to hospital for investigations. The blood test was repeated and a bone marrow biopsy was performed. Later that day John was told that he had acute myeloid leukaemia.

Chemotherapy was started immediately and John was isolated in a single room so that he could be protected as the treatment would make him vulnerable to infections. For the next six months John had intensive chemotherapy only being allowed home in between the treatments if his blood count had recovered sufficiently from the neutropenic period.

After the chemotherapy had been completed John had hoped that he would be cured. He had to return to the hospital for fortnightly and then weekly blood tests but unfortunately less than three months after finishing the treatment a blood test showed that the leukaemia had returned. He asked the specialist how long he had to live and she informed him between four to six months. John was understandably shocked.

John was then referred to a specialist centre for the treatment of leukaemia to see if they would consider treating him with a stem cell transplant. His GP warned that it wasn't very likely because 55 years was the limit as the treatment was so toxic to the body. John said, 'I knew I had got the dreaded leukaemia and that it kills and I also knew I was at the wrong age for them to spend thousands and thousands of pounds on a patient but I had a big ace up my sleeve – my twin brother James.' A bone marrow sample was taken from his James and tested and found to be a 100% match to John's own bone marrow. 'When the news came through I knew I had a second chance on life.' The decision was made to go ahead and treat John.

Having a complete bone marrow match meant that the after-effects of a stem cell transplant would be reduced. However, John was informed by the haematologists that he had a 20% chance of not surviving the treatment. This consisted of chemotherapy, whole body radiotherapy over two daily sessions for five days, and a stem cell transplant with the cells from his brother infused into John like a blood transfusion. John found that he suffered some very severe side-effects, especially acute sickness and diarrhoea, which lasted for about four weeks after the transplant. The worst thing was not being able to eat and drink because of the metallic taste everything had that passed through his lips. His skin became brown, his hair fell out, he lost weight and became very weak. John feels that will-power and determination helped him to recover.

It was when John went home after being in hospital for five and a half weeks that he gradually started to regain his strength and his appetite. He says, 'It was porridge and Weetabix that kept me alive.' Now he feels 90% back to normal. He is not so exhausted and he is trying to build up his muscles with exercise. He now has blood tests once a fortnight and sees the haematologist every two months – 'I always worry until I have the results of the blood test.' John feels his own strength and attitude helped him through the treatment and he never complained. 'I've laid there in bed and told myself that being 63, I'm a lucky person. There are a lot of people that have died at 5, 10, 15 years of age. Although all my plans for retirement came to an abrupt end I'm not really annoyed because I am alive and kicking.'

Where conventional cancer chemotherapy is unlikely to produce a cure, more powerful methods of treatment have to be found. Chief among these at present is the use of bone marrow transplantation, originally introduced for leukaemia, but now more widely used to increase dose intensity with an acceptable margin of safety for the patient.

bone marrow transplants

ALLOGENEIC TRANSPLANTATION
Patients with leukaemia undergo very intensive chemotherapy (sometimes with whole body irradiation as well) to deliberately suppress to the point of zero function (ablate) their bone marrow. Then transplantation of matched marrow, generally from a sibling, might safely be able to repopulate the recipient's marrow with the leukaemia completely destroyed by the high-dose chemo-radiotherapy. This is a more dangerous procedure than autologous transplantation (described below) but it is also more often curative.

AUTOLOGOUS TRANSPLANTATION
An alternative approach, both for leukaemia, lymphoma and even some of the solid tumours, is to remove part of the patient's own bone marrow, then give very high-dose chemotherapy (again, possibly with total body irradiation as well), finally returning the patient's own marrow once again. With this form of transplantation there is no risk of transplantation mis-match (after all, it's the patient's own marrow that is removed and then returned) and so potentially has very wide applications in cancer work. It could prove to be the most logical means of providing much higher doses with relative safety. In certain tumours, such as Hodgkin's disease, the non-Hodgkin's lymphomas and testicular tumours no longer responsive to conventional treatment but possibly suitable for experimental therapy, such techniques have produced cures where the patient would otherwise have died.

The use of autologous bone marrow transplantation has allowed oncologists to become much bolder in their choice of chemotherapy dosage, thus widening the potential of successful treatment for a far larger patient group.

BLOOD STEM CELL TRANSPLANTATION
Even more exciting is the development during the 1990s of peripheral blood stem cell (PBSC) transplantation, which has increasingly replaced autologous bone marrow transplantation. In this technique, the patient's bone marrow is stimulated either by low-dose chemotherapy or CSF-type cytokines to liberate early marrow precursor cells into the circulating blood. These can then be collected, concentrated and used as support for high-dose chemotherapy. The technique can be repeated and much higher doses of chemotherapy safely given. This may eventually prove an effective way forward in breast, lung and other common solid cancers, but the results of ongoing studies have to be looked at.

SUPPORTIVE CARE

Many of the standard cancer treatments currently available are undeniably tough on the patient. Whether or not he was the first to point it out, Shakespeare was surely right when he noted, *'Desperate diseases by desperate means are cur'd/Or not at all,'* and it is true, as already pointed out, that both radiotherapy and chemotherapy may have to be given intensively, with the possibility of unwelcome side-effects, to be effective. Perhaps Shakespeare missed his true vocation: he was a cancer physician manqué.

Since we are stuck with beneficial treatments that cause side-effects in quite a high proportion of patients, methods of alleviating these problems

PAM'S STORY

Pam's cancer was diagnosed five years ago when she was 55 years old. She has one son and has been a widow since her husband died in 1989. She lives in East Grinstead and has spent the majority of her life in the house where she grew up as a child.

Pam first recognised something was wrong when she had an ulcerated area in her mouth. She went to her GP but it was when she went to her dentist for a routine dental check the following week that she was referred to a local hospital. A biopsy of the ulcerated tissue was taken and the diagnosis of oral (mouth) cancer was made. Pam was admitted to hospital to have the tumour removed from her bottom gum. The following day she was referred for laser treatment – photo dynamic therapy. This treatment consists of a sensitising agent applied to the site of the tumour, then a laser of the appropriate wavelength is used to irradiate the area, which results in a breakdown of the sensitising agent into cytotoxic substances, resulting in destruction of the tumour cells.

Unfortunately, Pam then had a recurrence of the tumour, which again was confirmed by a biopsy. The tumour was large and radical surgery was required to remove the tumour and then to reconstruct the defect. This was performed a few days later. Pam's jaw bone was removed and a new jaw was created with bone taken from her hip and muscle from her breast. The surgeon's aim was to reduce physical disfigurement and loss of function and help to restore some ability to swallow and maintain intelligible speech.

As well as the distress caused to the patient by having cancer, people who have had head and neck surgery see themselves as changed; their identity and self-image has altered. Pam was shocked when she first looked in the mirror; her face was very swollen and she hardly recognised herself. After recovering from the surgery, Pam underwent six weeks of daily radiotherapy treatment as an outpatient. Once this treatment was completed Pam shut herself off from the outside world. She would not go out of her house. If she did venture out she found people would stare and she became very angry and upset at this . She says, 'I still get annoyed if people stare at me. I can say I never had any physical pain, only psychological pain from my appearance. This type of cancer is difficult, you have to deal with having cancer and also have to deal with how you look. When I look into the mirror it is not me I see. Most cancers can be hidden under clothing but with mouth cancer it cannot.' In the early days Pam would cover up her face with scarves – even in her house in case anyone came to the door – and she avoided looking in mirrors.

Pam found all this very hard to cope with. However, the most difficult aspect that she had to face was seeing her family, friends and colleagues and to have to deal with their reaction to how her looks had as far as possible have had to be found. During treatment, patients sometimes need a whole variety of supportive remedies to help them to get through the treatment in the safest possible way. In addition, of course, their psychological state of mind is bound to be disturbed, to say the least, and it can only be hoped that family, friends and professional counsellors can provide the reassurance, love and support that they require. Many patients find it comforting to know that they are not alone in their anguish and fears, and find self-help support groups, run by those who have been through the same thing themselves, at least as valuable as anything else (see useful addresses on page 216). This may not be suitable for all patients, but health care professionals such as the specialist nurses, radiographers and the wider multi-disciplinary team, are there to help, to support and to care for patients throughout their treatment.

changed. She was afraid of their reaction and did not want people to sympathise or feel sorry for her. The result was that she preferred to stay at home and avoid seeing anyone.

Pam was offered counselling and had this six months after the surgery, which she found helpful. In hindsight she feels she would have benefited from the counselling beginning just after the operation. She has since had further surgery to remove some bone that had become dislodged and also damaged by radiotherapy treatment.

Pam has undergone a great deal of treatment over the past five years, which has required her to cope, adjust and adapt. She is now feeling physically well and attends the maxillo-facial unit at the hospital for regular assessment. She has some dental problems, which the dental surgeon is helping to resolve, and she also has some eating difficulties, which at the moment means that she can only eat soft food and drink with a straw as part of her mouth is numb.

Recently Pam attended a patient support group to meet other patients who have been through a similar experience and she recognises how far she has come during the past five years. 'It made me feel proud that I am getting on with life – this has been a very long journey.' She has, however, decided not to go to any more support group sessions as she found the experience made her to start to think of the cancer again. She began to feel low and Pam says she wants to forget the experience as best she can and get on with her life. She says that it would have been useful to attend such a group five years ago but there wasn't one established then. Pam believes you have got to fight for your life and not feel sorry for yourself. She says, 'I am Pam until I look in the mirror but now I have much more 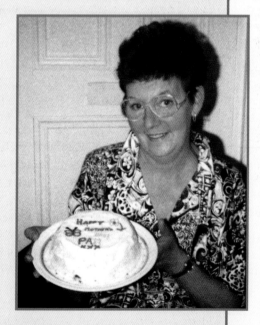 confidence in myself especially over the past six months. I know I will never look as I did, but this whole experience has made me stronger, I have coped and I am now getting on with my life. My goals are to stay healthy, carry on being happy, get a part-time job and to possibly have a tattoo!'

ONGOING CARE OPTIONS

Few diseases are associated with such fear and anxiety as cancer, since many of us assume that the disease will bring an inevitable progression of relentless new symptoms, uncontrollable suffering and certain death. One of the most difficult but rewarding tasks for the oncology team is to reassure patients that this is far from the truth, and to explain that cure or long-term remission is often possible. Although patients are better informed now than 20 years ago, partly as a result of wider discussion of cancer and its treatment within the media, medical knowledge, even among well-educated people, is often fragmentary and surprisingly incomplete. Doctors, too, can be disinclined to speak frankly with patients, and some may not have the communication skills

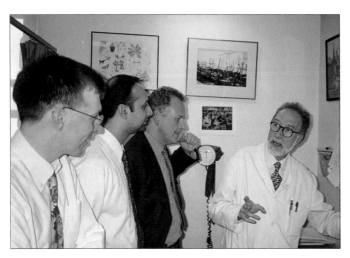

to do it very well. Specialists don't always realise that even a condition such as breast cancer is not all that common in a general practice setting, compared with far more frequently encountered benign disorders.

For all these reasons, the importance of communication between specialists, multi-disciplinary team, patients and general practitioners cannot be over-stressed. Communication is often the key to successful management of the most difficult problems of all, namely those in which cure is impossible and the outcome likely to be fatal. Special-ists in continuing and palliative care teams have often highlighted lack of communication as the greatest barrier to satisfactory supportive care during the patient's final six weeks. They point out that a 'good death' is a realistic possibility, particularly since, during this final phase, when active anti-cancer treatment is no longer possible, both the family and the patient have probably accepted the inevitable, at least in principle, to a greater degree than the doctors involved.

Part of our oncology team, meeting weekly for a pre-ward round discussion to try to work out the best treatment plan for each patient. With nursing staff, nutrition specialists, social workers and so on, the room can get pretty crowded.

continuing care options

'Continuing care' is a loose term that is often taken to mean the care of a cancer patient who is unlikely to be cured, who is not yet close to death, but who has certain physical and emotional needs. Increasingly it is recognised that these may well be not best served in the hospital setting, with its emphasis on acute and active care, action, noise, speedy recovery for others, and a chronic lack of time for medical and nursing staff to help the patient in the best possible way. For all these reasons, hospitals may be less than an ideal setting for cancer patients during the final weeks or months of life. For the most part, they simply don't need the high-tech services which have increasingly become the *raison d'être* for modern hospital in-patient care.

IN A HOSPICE

Hospices aim to provide special sanctuaries for patients like this who need a quite different environment – a calm setting instead of the usual ward buzz, with plenty of time for reflection and discussion with the staff, and a quite different set of priorities from

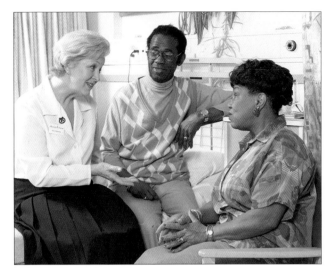

Specialists such as Macmillan nurses have a vital role to play in ongoing care for patient and family or friend.

that of the acute general hospital. The speed with which the hospice movement took root is clearly an indication of the scale of the need, and Britain can certainly claim pride of place in the development of what has now become a world-wide attack on inadequate standards of care. One real benefit has been, ironically, that the hospital environment has also improved considerably over the past decade, with much more attention now being given to proper control of pain and other symptoms. Patients at most large hospitals no longer have to 'earn' their pain killers in the way that used to be commonplace, not out of spite but generally the result of ignorance and an absurd and misplaced fear, by doctors and nurses alike, about addiction to strong opiate drugs, such as morphine.

AT HOME

Increasingly, cancer patients, whether curable or not, are looked after in the community, often with the aid of Macmillan or Marie Curie nurses who are specially trained in supportive care and generally highly skilled. Alternatively, there is the support of a multi-disciplinary team comprising nursing staff, social workers and doctors. The development of these teams has resulted in far better care for cancer patients throughout the country than would have been dreamed possible even ten years ago, and most areas now have them. They offer highly specialised advice about the choice and scheduling of pain drugs for cancer, and the prevention and treatment of side-effects.

Agents such as morphine can be quite difficult to handle. All strong pain killers, for example, tend to constipate, and it is extremely important to warn patients about this and to give the appropriate laxative when starting opiates for the first time. This applies not only to morphine, but to all codeine derivatives (particularly the commonly used dihydrocodeine or DF118) (see page 213).

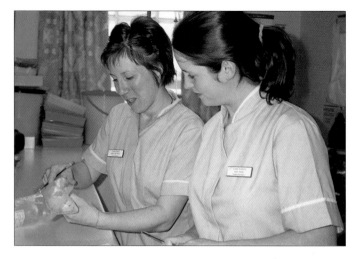

Checking of chemotherapy for infusion is an essential part of the routine of oncology departments.

Multi-disciplinary teams often provide the best links between specialist and GP, visiting the patient as required, on a regular basis both at home and in hospital. They can help with choosing the best time for the patient's discharge from hospital, bearing in mind the support the patient has at home and any particular needs. These might include having a modified bathroom with supportive rails and wheelchair access, or the transfer of a bedroom from an upper to a lower floor. The support team is also very likely to have built a closer relationship with family members than would have been possible in hospital, involving a spouse or partner in the patient's recovery, particularly if a major operation, such as mastectomy or radical hysterectomy, has been necessary.

how long have I got?

As pointed out by Dr Maurice Slevin, chairman of the patient organisation CancerBACUP (British Association of Cancer United Patients):

'It is almost always negative to tell people that they have a fixed life expectancy. The averages apply to populations and not to individuals, and to give people a fixed life expectancy removes hope and provokes depression and despondency. It is more appropriate and helpful to indicate that, while life might be very short if things go badly, the length of life could still be long and cannot be estimated if things go well.'

The truth, of course, is that all medical practitioners, even specialists, are pretty imprecise when it comes to measuring the likely survival of a patient who can't be cured. In this respect, they are generally wide of the mark. One study discovered, for example, that most doctors' predictions were too long, probably because of their innate optimism. Some patients, however, do wish to be told a certain length of time, perhaps to put their affairs in order or to make a special trip, and this of course poses a particular difficulty. It is usually better to provide an 'envelope' of time, rather than make a specific guess, which is so likely to be wrong. It might seem a sensible idea to suggest a time interval which, on the face of it, is rather shorter than the doctor's genuine belief (partly on the grounds that patients gain considerable satisfaction from living longer than the doctor predicted), but this can be seen as a harsh approach, and, on the whole, perhaps it's better to express genuine uncertainty. One further problem comes with the strong request from a family member to be silent (or frankly mendacious), even if the patient him- or herself puts pointed questions about longevity. This really does put the doctor on the spot.

As Professor Souhami writes in his book *Cancer and its Management* (co-authored with Dr Tobias), 'There are few other branches of medicine which demand simultaneously such technical expertise and kindly understanding as does cancer medicine. The strains on the doctor are considerable, especially if he takes the human aspect of his work seriously. It is a great failing in a doctor if he talks to his patients only about the physical and technical aspects of the illness, relies heavily on investigation in making treatment decisions and finds it difficult to give up intensive measures and accept that the patient cannot be cured. Technical prowess is then replaced by thoughtful analysis of the patient's feelings and what is in his best interest.

'Treating patients with cancer demands great resources of emotional energy on the part of the doctor. In some units, part of the work of talking to patients is taken over by psychiatrists, psychologists, social workers or other counsellors. Invaluable though help from these persons may be, we do not think it desirable that doctors should see themselves as technical experts and that, when human feelings intrude into the medical situation, the patient should be sent to talk to someone else about their problems. Sustaining and supporting a patient and his relatives is a matter of teamwork, but the doctor in charge of the case must make it clear that he or she regards the psychological aspects of the disease to be as important as the physical.'

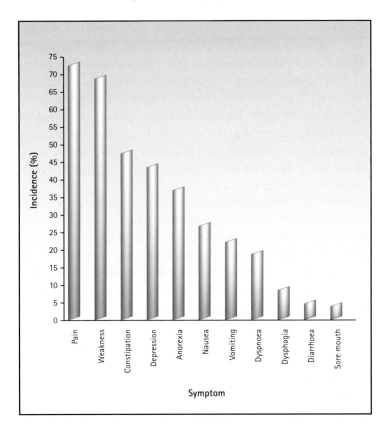

Common symptoms in cancer. These are very approximate figures but give a useful indication of problems that may be encountered. All of them – without exception – can be treated, often with great benefit. Attention to detail is essential.

PAIN AND SYMPTOM CONTROL

The fear of unremitting pain as the cancer progresses, traditionally voiced by so many cancer patients, should for the most part be a thing of the past (see boxes, left and opposite). There is a sufficient choice of versatile drugs for adequate pain relief to be possible in almost all cases, though considerable skill is required in order to achieve this. The use of regular, rather than 'as required' pain relief, together with laxatives, steroids, anti-depressants and so on, together with supportive drugs, has made an immense difference. Without wishing to appear too messianic, there really shouldn't be an excuse any longer for doctors to be overcautious about increasing dosage, particularly of morphine, to the level required for adequate pain relief. One of the remarkable features of morphine as a pharmacological agent is its very wide spectrum of dose, probably wider than any other drug in use. Some patients require 30 milligrams twice daily of the commonly prescribed, long-acting tablets containing morphine sulphate, others ten times this or even more. The availability of the long-acting (12-hour) preparation has made patients' lives very much easier, since they no longer have to cart around large bottles of morphine elixir. The majority now live comfortable and sometimes surprisingly normal lives, frequently continuing this way – and deriving enormous psychological satisfaction from it – until shortly before death. It's best to keep the pain prescriptions simple:

• For mild or moderate cancer pain, aspirin, paracetamol and co-proxamol (Distalgesic) are all helpful, and the first two, of course, can be purchased without a medical prescription. Anti-inflammatory agents, such as ibuprofen (now available in 200 milligram strength without prescription) are often also helpful. Other useful drugs in this group are diclofenac (Voltarol) and naproxen (Naprosyn).

• For stronger pain relief, codeine and its derivatives are often prescribed, but are extremely constipating. This is such a demoralising and sometimes painful problem that it really is important to prevent it occurring in the first place. If the doctor doesn't prescribe a laxative when offering codeine or dihydrocodeine for the first time, ask for one – you'll probably need it.

• For severe or stubborn cancer pain, there really is no better drug than morphine. It's not uncommon for patients to have been on lesser remedies for far too long before switching over; the sense of relief and improvement in their well-being is almost palpable. Long-acting morphine preparations have revolutionised cancer care. Patients don't seem to need an inevitable increase in dosage anything like as quickly as might be imagined. Addiction simply isn't a problem, so the dose should be whatever is required to give adequate pain relief. One of the greatest benefits of adequate morphine is the enormous improvement in quality of sleep, often for the first time after months of demoralising discomfort. If necessary, strong pain killers can also be given by injection, skin patch or as suppositories. By mouth is usually best, though.

Another extremely important symptom of advanced cancer is the loss of appetite (often termed 'anorexia') so commonly experienced as the cancer progresses. 'How's your appetite?' is often the most useful and revealing of all the questions during this later stage. A number of factors contribute to this important symptom (see box, below) and several agents, particularly cortisone and similar drugs, can be helpful. Small meals are often more acceptable. It may be beneficial to see a dietician for advice. Above all else, it is never right for a doctor to shrug his or her shoulders and claim there is nothing more he or she can do. It is quite wrong for patients to be abandoned in this way; indeed, patients often make a far less clear-cut distinction between active and passive treatment than doctors do, and are generally extremely appreciative of the doctor's attempts to get the details of pain and symptom control right. It's not the gratitude that's important, of course, but the implication that to the patient these details really do matter.

There can't, of course, be any simple solution to the best means of providing social support and symptomatic care during the final weeks or months of life. Circumstances vary so widely. But the increasing recognition that widespread cancer is not a diagnosis that needs to be stigmatised or pushed aside has helped immeasurably. So, too, has the wider application of the many principles of supportive care outlined on the previous pages. With proper attention to detail, the right type of medication, adequate local resources and frequent review many more patients can be helped so that 'death with dignity' becomes more than a hollow and unfulfilled promise.

MILD, MODERATE AND POWERFUL ANALGESICS USED FOR PAIN RELIEF

A cancer sufferer should first be maintained on mild analgesics until the maximum recommended dose fails to control pain. They are then moved on to a moderate analgesic, until once again the maximum recommended dose fails. They then progress to a powerful analgesic.

Non-steroidal anti-inflammatory drugs
Aspirin
Paracetamol
Naproxen

Compound analgesics
Co-proxamol
Co-dydramol
Co-codamol

Morphine and other opiates
Morphine sulphate
Diamorphine hydrochloride
Oxycodone pectinate

FACTORS CONTRIBUTING TO WEIGHT LOSS

FACTOR	CAUSE
Anorexia, nausea and vomiting	Tumour
	Treatment
	Psychological factors (pain and depression)
Loss of protein, blood and minerals	Diarrhoea
	Ulceration
	Bleeding
Malabsorption and intestinal obstruction	Carcinoma of pancreas and ovary
Metabolic abnormalities induced by the tumour insulin resistance	Increased protein breakdown, metabolic rate or fat breakdown
	Altered glucose metabolism due to increased lactate recycling or
	Tumour metabolism of protein and carbohydrate
External influences	Chemotherapy (nausea, vomiting, mucositis)
	Radiotherapy (nausea, vomiting, diarrhoea)

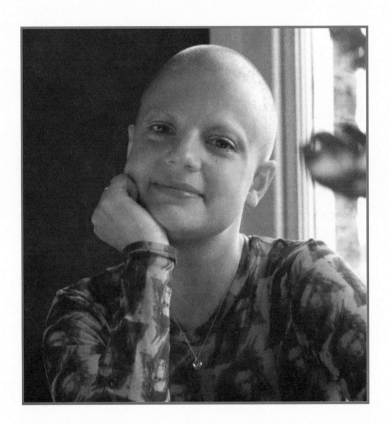

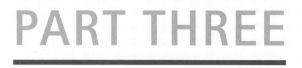

PART THREE

TYPES OF CANCER

❛ It was a release to get a diagnosis – cancer knocks you for six, facing this illness. It makes you re-evaluate everything; what you do with your time, how you see other people, and how you see the things you do. It really has shifted my perspective on a lot of things and the way I look at things and how I live my life now. ❜

GLEN XAVIER

THE MOST COMMON CANCERS

LUNG CANCER

Lung cancer represents one of the greatest tragedies of the Western world, summed up in an old *Punch* cartoon, which shows Sir Walter Raleigh talking to his mate when they discover tobacco for the first time; the friend is saying, *'Well, don't worry, Walt; if we discover it's dangerous, we can always give it up.'*

causes

Lung cancer is by far the most common cancer in the West, having increased steadily in incidence since the 1930s and possibly just beginning to dip. Cigarette smoking became popular in the trenches in the First World War, and we now know that the epidemic of lung cancer, wherever in the world you look at it, follows the introduction of cigarette smoking by about 20 years. This is equally true for women, who started to take up smoking in large numbers in the 1950s, just as men did 30 years before. The link between cigarette smoking and lung cancer is absolutely clear cut, just as it is known that stopping smoking is most certainly followed by a reduction in the individual's risk of developing lung cancer. After about 15 years of non-smoking, the risk is almost as low as if the individual had never smoked at all (see box, left).

There is no doubt that the tobacco industry has successfully targeted young people and women. In the 1950s, the male-to-female ratio for lung cancer was over ten to one, i.e. women formed less than 10% of the total, but by 1984, the figure stood at only four to one (i.e. 25% of all lung cancer cases were now women). The gap has closed even further since then (in 1997 it was about two to one). Smoking habits are closely linked to socio-economic group. In some parts of the UK, particularly in Scotland, lung cancer in women has overtaken breast cancer as the most common of all female cancers.

Recent debate has centred on the dangers of passive smoking, and it is now known that non-smoking women who are married to smokers face a risk of lung cancer which is over twice what it would be if they (as non-smokers) were married to men who also did not smoke. A few years ago the Royal College of Physicians issued a devastating report on the dangers of passive smoking in children, including the probability of an increased risk of cot death, asthma and other childhood diseases. In Britain, cigarettes are now relatively cheaper than they were 25 years ago, and restriction of smoking in public areas has been a protracted and uphill battle. The death rate from this disease remains extremely high, since it is both common and, in most cases, very difficult to cure. On its own, lung cancer accounts for about a quarter of all cancer deaths in Britain each year.

THE RISK OF SMOKERS DEVELOPING LUNG CANCER

• Risk is directly related to the number of cigarettes smoked, i.e. the higher the consumption, the higher the risk.

• Risk is more dependent on duration of smoking than on consumption, e.g. smoking one packet of cigarettes a day for 40 years is eight times more hazardous than smoking two packets a day for 20 years.

• If you stop smoking, the risk is definitely reduced. Smokers who stop before the age of 35 years have an expectation of life not significantly different from non-smokers, while stopping in middle age before the onset of cancer or some other serious disease avoids most of the later excess risk from tobacco.

Other causes of lung cancer pale into insignificance when compared with cigarette smoking, at least in the Western world. In the Middle and Far East and other areas of the developing world, lung cancer is emerging as a major health hazard, just as in the West. These countries face a tremendous struggle against the self-promotion of a powerful and sophisticated tobacco industry, unrestrained by governmental and social pressures, which now operate more effectively in the West.

That is not to say that there are grounds for complacency here at home. Although a no-smoking policy now operates in many public places, on public transport and so on, the rates of incidence and mortality from lung cancer are falling only slowly, and, in some social groups, barely at all. There is no proof as yet that low-tar brands, now very actively advertised, are necessarily safer than traditional ones, or that the government health warnings seen on hoardings and cigarette packs are all that effective. Many believe that a total ban on tobacco advertising would be far preferable, particularly since children and young people can all too easily obtain cigarettes and fall prey to a habit that will dent their finances, clog their heart and lungs, stain their teeth, make them and their clothes smelly and unappealing, and, in the end, quite possibly prove fatal. The cost of treating cigarette-related diseases (the cost to all of us, that is, since most of us are taxpayers) is enormous, particularly since chronic heart and lung disease may persist for years before the death of the patient. If cigarette smoking had never been invented, so to speak, what is today our most common cancer would be something of a medical rarity. Instead of which, we have an epidemic of horrendous proportions:

● Patients who smoke 10 to 20 a day have a risk of lung cancer 30 times greater than non-smokers.

● For people who smoke 40 a day the risk is 60 times greater.

● Nearly 40,000 people in Britain develop lung cancer each year, and over 90% die from it, usually within two years. Many are in their fifties and sixties.

● Of the other risk factors only asbestos and air pollution are seriously worth considering, though these are far less important.

Since lung cancer is so difficult to cure, and so damaging in its effects before death, the importance of cutting down or, better still, stopping smoking cannot be overstressed. The only time to do it is now!

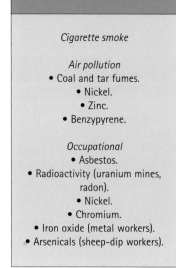

KNOWN CAUSES OF LUNG CANCER

Cigarette smoke

Air pollution
● Coal and tar fumes.
● Nickel.
● Zinc.
● Benzypyrene.

Occupational
● Asbestos.
● Radioactivity (uranium mines, radon).
● Nickel.
● Chromium.
● Iron oxide (metal workers).
● Arsenicals (sheep-dip workers).

types of lung cancer

There are many types of lung cancer, which are divided into two main groups: non-small-cell carcinomas, which comprise squamous cell carcinomas, adenocarcinomas and large-cell carcinomas, and small-cell carcinomas. The three cancers in the non-small-cell lung cancer group are often regarded jointly for treatment purposes since the medical management is similar for each, and quite different from what is recommended for small-cell lung cancer.

Non-small-cell lung cancer: Squamous cell carcinoma (see page 28) is the most common form of lung cancer, generally arising from one of the main bronchi, the major pathway from the trachea, or windpipe, to the lungs themselves. This type of tumour accounts for over half of the cases seen in Britain and is exceptionally rare in non-smokers. Adenocarcinoma (see page 28) is the less common variety of lung cancer, it is far less closely linked with cigarette smoking.

Small-cell lung cancer: Pathologically and in its natural history this type is a quite different entity and is even rarer in non-smokers. It may look the same as a squamous cell carcinoma on a chest X-ray but in reality, it is even more lethal, with very rapid spread to other parts of the body, and a high rate of malignant cell division. This makes it the most rapidly fatal of all the lung cancers, with a very poor cure rate, despite a high initial response rate to treatment (see page 73).

symptoms and diagnosis

Typical symptoms in lung cancer patients include:
- Coughing, often with bloodstained sputum.
- Shortness of breath.
- Chest pain.
- Many patients will be used to at least some of these symptoms since smokers frequently develop chronic bronchitis and have come to expect winter exacerbations. However, in patients with lung cancer, the symptoms are often more severe, and the sputum may be bloodstained for the first time.
- Some patients develop a pneumonia which is slow to resolve despite antibiotics, and a few will have difficulties in swallowing because of the compression of the oesophagus caused by enlarged cancerous glands in the chest.
- Many patients will have lost weight, and will have become increasingly uninterested in food.
- Others will turn up for the first time, not with complaints relating to the primary tumour but, bearing in mind the frequency with which lung cancers spread to other parts of the body, with symptoms from this secondary spread. This might include, for example, severe pain or even a fracture of a long bone or vertebra from a secondary bone deposit; sudden loss of function of an arm or leg from a secondary (often multiple) in the brain; or the patient may have noticed an enlarged gland in the neck that turns out to be an obviously involved lymph node.

DIAGNOSIS

Diagnosis is usually straightforward. Most lung cancers are visible on a chest X-ray, and confirmation of an abnormal shadow can usually be obtained either by examination of sputum under the microscope or by a technique known as bronchoscopy, in which a semi-flexible fibre-optic tube is passed, under a light anaesthetic, through the nose, larynx and windpipe, down the bronchial passages to the site of the abnormality. The physician can then take a small biopsy under direct vision – in most cases of lung cancer, the malignant ulcer will be easily visible.

Lung cancers are among the most dangerous and lethal of all, since they can spread so widely – particularly the small-cell variety. Potential secondary sites include liver, brain, long bones and vertebrae, skin, lymph nodes and intra-abdominal soft tissues – almost anywhere, in fact. For these reasons, surgical removal of a lung cancer, so valuable in a minority of patients, cannot always be relied upon.

treatment

Which brings us to treatment. There is no doubt that, wherever possible, a lung cancer should be surgically removed, since this technique has the greatest chance of long-term success. The trouble is that only a smallish minority of lung cancer cases are really suitable for surgery (see box, opposite). In the first place, all the small-cell lung cancer cases (about 25% of the total) are surgically out of bounds, since they are so likely to have spread well beyond the primary site. This is generally the case even where exhaustive scanning and other investigations don't show obvious secondary deposits outside the chest. Surgery for these patients just makes things worse.

NON-SMALL-CELL LUNG CANCER

Surgery: In the non-small-cell cancer group, surgery is well worth considering and will be recommended if the patient fulfils certain criteria. For one thing, the tumour cannot be situated too close to the centre of the chest, since the closer it lies to the point of division of the two main bronchi from the windpipe, the less possible it is for the surgeon to clear the tumour, even by removing the whole of the lung. The more peripherally placed the tumour (i.e. the further out towards the edge of the lung) the more operable it will be. Surgeons and patients would much prefer to remove part of the lung – the lobe in which the tumour is situated – than remove the whole lung itself, as the functional consequences are far less severe. The general condition of the patient must, of course, be pretty good, since many have been heavy smokers and may be suffering from bronchitis or heart disease, which could make them unsuitable for surgery even if they have an operable tumour. Some patients have a collection of fluid below the lung, which is likely to contain malignant cells (a malignant plural effusion), which again counts against them as far as operability is concerned, since these patients have an unacceptable probability of local tumour occurrence after surgery. And so on.

Radiotherapy: For patients with non-small-cell lung cancer who are inoperable for any of these reasons, radiotherapy is worth considering,

MARY'S STORY

Mary had always been a heavy smoker – she admitted to 40 a day, but her husband said it was nearer sixty. She was 54 when she was admitted to hospital. She was brought into casualty late on a Friday evening after closing time, severely breathless and with a handkerchief full of blood clot. Like so many patients with lung cancer, she'd suddenly gone off cigarettes entirely, after smoking about a quarter of a million of them during her lifetime. The chest X-ray showed complete collapse of the right lung, so no wonder she was breathless. The chest team did the bronchoscopy and saw a large tumour sitting only 2 centimetres beyond the point where the windpipe divides into the right and left main bronchi. It turned out to be a small-cell cancer, best treated by chemotherapy.

She was treated within a chemo-radiation trial and a month of radiation therapy to the chest. Although it never returned to normal, the chest X-ray dramatically improved, and her lung re-inflated. Four months later, however, a gland appeared in her neck. A needle biopsy confirmed the worst. 'How could it have come back so fast?' asked her husband. Like most patients with small-cell lung cancer, Mary's tumour, though so responsive the first time round, proved almost fully resistant to chemotherapy on the second occasion. After two courses of chemotherapy using newer drugs not included in the initial choice, it was clear that she was getting nowhere. Local radiotherapy to the neck was successful in shrinking down the glandular mass, but within a further two months, Mary had developed secondary deposits in the liver, ribs and skin. 'Surely there must be something more that you can do?' her husband asked the consultant. Sadly, there wasn't.

Small-cell lung cancer has a very poor prognosis, all the more tragic since it is so closely related to cigarette smoking and would be a rare condition if smoking had never been invented, so to speak. However, not all patients with lung cancer do so poorly. Patients with operable cancers (always of the non-small-cell variety) have a real chance of cure (see overleaf).

but in truth is likely to be more valuable for palliation of symptoms rather than as a treatment with a real prospect of cure. For symptoms such as coughing up blood, chest pain, obstruction of a large-bore bronchial pathway or swallowing difficulty from nodal enlargement pressing on the gullet, radiotherapy may be extremely valuable, but there's no point in taxing the patient with a very high dose of radiotherapy in the hope of cure, since a cure couldn't realistically be attempted, except very occasionally in patients who fulfil all the criteria for operability, but either turn down an operation (some do, surprisingly) or have another serious condition, which makes the anaesthetic too risky.

There are particular situations where radiotherapy can be really valuable. As a result of direct pressure from the cancer, some patients develop a life-threatening degree of obstruction of the main blood vessel (superior vena cava), which returns blood from the upper half of the body. This syndrome of superior vena cava obstruction can cause tremendous pressure in the face and neck, with a bloated, bluish appearance and strikingly visible distended veins in the neck. Although extremely serious if left untreated, radiotherapy often provides quick and quite effective relief. In other sites within the chest, direct pressure from the primary tumour or enlarged glands can cause collapse of all or part of the lung. Radiotherapy can shrink these masses, often successfully re-inflating the lung again. Other important clinical syndromes in lung cancer include loss of voice from erosion of the laryngeal nerve by a tumour mass deep in the chest, or destruction of the upper chest wall and ribs, with severe shoulder pain and arm weakness by a tumour situated at the lung apex.

Chemotherapy: This is emerging as a genuinely valuable form of treatment in non-small-cell lung cancer, though there is no agreement so far among professionals as to the best drug combinations. Most are based on cisplatin, and NICE (the National Institute for Clinical Excellence) has recently approved several other new drugs as well, including gemcitabine, paclitaxel and vinorelbine.

SMALL-CELL LUNG CANCER

Chemotherapy: In small-cell lung cancer, the treatment is different because surgery is never sufficient (and therefore not worth doing at all). Both chemotherapy and radiation are far more appropriate. Small-cell lung cancer usually responds to chemotherapy to a striking degree, though to the clinician this is one of the most frustrating of tumours since the early dramatic response to chemotherapy is rarely beyond a year or two. It is not uncommon to share with the patient the joy of seeing the chest X-ray return to normal, only to point out grimly, perhaps six months later, the equally clear evidence of the return of the cancer, with far fewer treatment options the second time around.

Combined chemotherapy and radiation: There is no clear advantage for one type of chemotherapy over another; but one recent improvement, at least for patients with 'limited disease', i.e. with the tumour confined to the chest, without evidence of spread, has been the use of combined chemotherapy and radiotherapy to the chest, a treatment approach now known to be more beneficial than the use of chemotherapy alone. It's more taxing too, with side-effects such as swallowing difficulty from inflammation of the oesophagus and skin discomfort within the irradiated area. Radiotherapy alone, without chemotherapy, isn't used for small-cell lung cancer (apart from patients who are felt to be too unwell to cope with chemotherapy), since this form of treatment would miss any opportunity for control of secondary tumours at other sites.

prognosis

There's no getting away from the fact that the outlook in lung cancer is generally poor. Patients who are suitable for surgical treatment are in a fortunate minority, and some surgeons claim long-term cure rates in

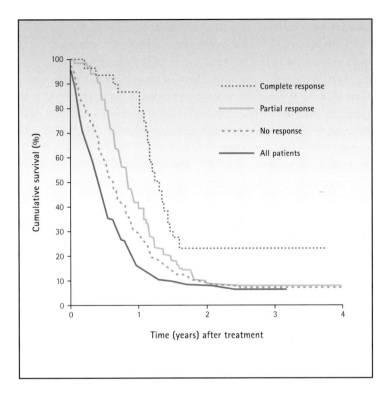

Survival and response rates to combination chemotherapy (small-cell lung cancer).

as many as 50% of such cases. Sadly, however, very few of the inoperable group of long-term patients are curable, apart from a small group with small-cell lung cancer where there is no evidence of spread beyond the chest (10% at the most) who respond dramatically and durably to chemotherapy treatment.

NON-SMALL-CELL LUNG CANCER

Patients with non-small-cell lung cancer occasionally do well, long term, with radical radiotherapy. Recent studies suggest that chemotherapy may turn out to be modestly beneficial, too. Trial groups both in the UK and elsewhere are trying as best they can to pursue some randomised studies, which are the only means of settling this question for sure.

SMALL-CELL LUNG CANCER

In small-cell lung cancer, the frustrating paradox is that this tumour is so readily responsive to chemotherapy, at least in the first instance, yet overall has the worst outlook of any lung cancer type, with a very poor secondary response to chemotherapy (i.e. at relapse) despite the initial benefits that chemotherapy had achieved.

For patients with secondary spread from a lung cancer, radiotherapy is once again the most valuable form of treatment, particularly with bone secondaries. This is equally true for the small-cell and non-small-cell varieties.

GYNAECOLOGICAL CANCERS

World-wide, gynaecological cancers form a large and important group of illnesses. In parts of Asia and South America, cancer of the cervix, for example, is the most important cause of cancer mortality in women, though in Europe and North America, education and screening programmes have reduced the incidence and mortality very substantially. By contrast, the most serious threat in Europe and North America comes from ovarian carcinoma, which even now tends to be diagnosed at a relatively advanced stage and has a mortality rate equal to the combined mortality from cancers of the cervix and uterus combined.

Quite a lot is known about the causes of at least some of the major gynaecological cancers.

causes

CAUSES OF OVARIAN CANCER

● Women who have never been pregnant have an increased risk of developing the disease.

● It is also known that groups of women with low incidence, such as the Japanese, do quite rapidly increase their risk if they migrate to a Western society, such as the USA. A striking, fivefold increase seems to occur within a couple of generations, suggesting that environmental influences (rather than genetic ones) are likely to be the cause.

● Europe and the USA have the highest inci-

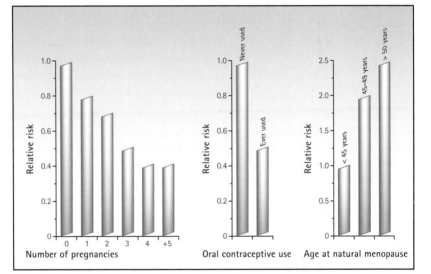

dence in the world, and there are certainly a number of families in which clusters of women with ovarian cancer have been identified.

For the most part, though, it seems to arise sporadically, though there is a weak linkage with breast cancer – possibly operating through the feature of sub-fertility, which is known to be a risk factor in both these conditions.

Clues to causation in ovarian cancer: relative risk rates with the number of pregnancies, use of the oral contraceptive and age at natural menopause.

CAUSES OF CERVICAL CANCER

● In cancer of the cervix, there is no doubt that sexual activity is very closely related, and it is now fairly clear that the cause of the illness is in an infectious virus or particle, the human papilloma virus.

GYNAECOLOGICAL CANCER
KEY POINTS

Ovarian cancer
- 5,400 cases each year in England and Wales.
- Uncommon below 40 years (5%).
- Symptoms – often vague/non-specific abdominal symptoms.
- 90% have a palpable pelvic mass.
- Usually diagnosed late.

Endometrial cancer
- 3,900 cases each year in England and Wales.
- Most patients (95%) present with postmenopausal bleeding.
- Uncommon in premenopausal women (less than 5%).

Cervical cancer
- 3,400 cases each year.
- Incidence similar across all age groups over 30 years of age.
- Screen programme aims to identify precursor lesions.
- Typical symptoms are postmenopausal, postcoital and persistent intermenstrual bleeding.
- Usually (80%) diagnosed on speculum examination.
- Up to 40% are screen detected.
- Any clinical suspicion is an indication for referral and not for a cervical smear.

- The risk of the most common type of cancer of the cervix (squamous cell carcinoma – see page 28) is unknown in nuns and other women who are lifelong celibates.
- There also seems to be a lowered risk in women who have had one or few sexual partners.
- The risk of disease seems particularly closely related to the age at which a woman's sexual activity first began – the lower the age, the higher the incidence. One explanation may well be that the developing immature epithelium (covering) of the cervix may be particularly susceptible during the immediate post-pubertal years to malign influences such as a virus particle, which might be acquired during intercourse.
- There are a few cases on record of couples who develop symptoms more or less simultaneously, with the male partner developing a carcinoma of the penis, and within a few years either side, the female partner or spouse developing a carcinoma of the cervix.
- For many years, it was suggested that intercourse only with circumcised men led to a lower incidence of cervical cancer, but this has been increasingly questioned.

Over the past 30 years, the peak age of incidence of cancer of the cervix has fallen, presumably because of changing sexual habits, but the good news is that an increasing proportion of tumours are diagnosed by cervical screening programmes while still in the pre-invasive and fully curable stage. Routine use of a barrier method of contraception (such as a condom) reduces the risk, again supporting the hypothesis that there is a transmissable agent acquired during intercourse and likely to be the cause. It is not a simple relationship, however, unlike, for example, the bacteria causing pneumonia or meningitis, or the viruses that cause mumps or chicken pox. The development of a malignant change is a very much slower process, and the causative events much harder to pin down because of the inevitable lag period from initial exposure to development of the disorder. Papilloma viruses are also known to cause genital warts, which seem to co-exist with pre-malignant cancer.

CAUSES OF UTERINE CANCER

In contrast to cancers of the cervix, these are most commonly adenocarcinomas and there are again wide variations in incidence across the world. It is much more common in Britain and the USA than West Africa, and in general is chiefly prevalent in the Western world.
- It is very much more common in grossly overweight (obese) women.
- To a lesser extent, it appears in patients with diabetes and hypertension.
- The highest rate of all is in the USA, where obesity has become a relatively common health problem. In large ladies with greater than normal fat stores, the normal circulating oestrogen is supplemented by the conversion of oestrogen precursors in these fat stores, effectively increasing the total circulating oestrogen level, so that stimulation (hyperplasia) of the uterine lining may take place. This development

can, on occasion, develop further, leading to cancer.

● Late menopause also seems to be a clear risk factor, again suggesting a common mechanism, since these patients have higher oestrogen levels over a longer period than normal.

Which brings us to the question of hormone replacement therapy (HRT). How safe is it? The generally accepted view is that modern types of HRT are extremely safe, since cyclical oestrogen/progesterone (either by mouth or patches) is recommended to mimic as far as possible the normal monthly human cycle. Avoiding over-exposure to high doses of oestrogens (often termed 'unopposed' oestrogens) is the key to reducing potential risks and there is no doubt that for many women the benefits of HRT (improved well-being and libido together with avoidance of osteoporosis and heart disease) greatly outweigh potential disadvantages. Women who have had a hysterectomy are at no risk of developing uterine carcinoma, so in these patients it is unnecessary to give progesterone-containing forms of HRT. Worries do persist, however, that the very widespread use of HRT, particularly with so many of us becoming increasingly overweight, may lead to an increase in uterine hyperplasia, with its theoretical danger of a small risk of

THE VALUE OF A REGULAR SMEAR TEST

In patients who are developing a true (invasive) cancer of the cervix, there is a clear development of cellular changes from normality through to an atypical (but not yet malignant) appearance (dysplasia), and then to various degrees of recognisable pre-malignant change (often known as carcinoma-in-situ or CIN). Not all patients with CIN will develop an invasive cancer, even without treatment, but a steady slow progression appears to occur in the majority.

In well-organised screening programmes, the cervical smear test is designed to make a definitive diagnosis of pre-cancerous abnormalities whilst they are still at this dysplastic or CIN stage. A regular smear check reliably supplies plenty of cells which are fixed directly on the microscope slide, to be identified by an experienced pathologist. The smear test (often called a Pap smear, after its inventor, Dr Papanicolaou) only takes a couple of minutes and can be carried out by a GP or a nurse at well woman or family planning clinics. Early treatment of dysplasia or even severe CIN changes (often referred to as CIN 3, the highest grade) should be 100% successful. Cervical screening should start early, shortly after a woman becomes sexually active, though government guidelines in the UK lag behind this. It should be repeated every two years, more frequently if dysplastic cells are encountered.

Despite the occasional highly publicised fault in our screening system, there is no doubt that the introduction of screening has led to a dramatic fall in the death rates from cervical cancer. Many cases, particularly in younger women, are now detected earlier at the pre-invasive stage when the disease poses little threat (at least to life, and generally not to fertility either). This is remarkable since, with increasing evidence of earlier sexual activity, and probably an increased number of partners as well, the stage in postwar Britain (and the West generally) was surely set for an increase in incidence and therefore mortality as well. Recent accounts of incompetent technique or false reporting clearly highlight the need for extreme vigilance at all stages of the screening process.

development of a malignant change. It seems sensible to recommend as low a dose of oestrogen as possible, most manufacturers of HRT preparations now providing more than one dose strength.

Fortunately, uterine cancer is one of the most curable forms of all human malignant disease (at least in most cases), but high-risk women (those who are grossly overweight, particularly if they have hypertension or diabetes, and are still menstruating over the age of 53), should be encouraged to lose weight and take proper advice to control the diabetes or high blood pressure as effectively as possible.

CAUSES OF VULVAL AND VAGINAL CANCERS

Cancers can occur in the lower parts of the female genital tract as well – the vulva and, much less commonly, the vagina. Vulval cancer is almost exclusively a disease of older women, above the age of 65, although exceptions do of course occur. As with cancers of the cervix, these are generally squamous cell carcinomas, and this is sometimes preceded, often over many years, by generalised skin changes (again, the term 'dysplastic' is often used, meaning a change in the normal cellular pattern of the skin). Just as with cancer of the cervix, some patients have evidence of carcinoma-in-situ, a pre-invasive condition, prior to developing the cancer. Itching, discomfort and occasional surface bleeding are all symptoms of this condition, though it is important to stress that benign causes of these symptoms are very much more common, candida infection, or thrush, being the most common of all.

symptoms and diagnosis

The symptoms of gynaecological cancer vary with the primary site. The lower female genital tract (vulva, vagina and visible part of the cervix) are positioned so low in the pelvis and are so accessible that symptoms usually occur early, in sharp contrast to cancers of the ovary.

● **Cancer of the vulva** (pretty unusual, only about a thousand new cases occurring annually in Britain) is generally accompanied by itching, pain, a lump on the labia, which the patient can feel herself, or a visible ulcer, sometimes with crust and a discharge. Anyone with problems of this type should obviously see their doctor, however embarrassed or sensitive they may be about it. Early treatment is the key to success.
● If these findings are associated with a lump in the groin area, rapid treatment is important, since the lump could either be a simple infected gland, or, much more seriously, a malignant lymph node.

● **Cancer of the cervix** is much more common, and the important symptoms are a persistent vaginal discharge, particularly if offensive (smelly) or bloodstained; and pain with intercourse or bleeding, particularly after sex.

● The larger and more locally advanced the tumour, the more obvious these symptoms are likely to be. Unfortunately, some women regard vaginal discharge or intermittent spotting bleeding as normal, and minimise the symptoms.

● Pre-invasive disease (dysplasia and CIN) are not usually associated with symptoms at all, but picked up by routine screening.

● **With uterine cancer**, the most common symptom is post-menopausal bleeding, and even a single episode should be taken seriously. About one-fifth of patients with uterine cancer are pre-menopausal, so bleeding between the periods is also important as a clinical symptom in younger women.

● **Ovarian cancer symptoms** are much more difficult to pin down and are frequently not very specific. The most common are lower abdominal pain, bloating, distension and loss of appetite, sometimes with nausea or bowel change. But these are such common symptoms in the normal population anyway that a GP almost has to develop superhuman skills to think of the diagnosis, let alone order the appropriate investigations or make a referral to a specialist on what are likely to seem rather spurious grounds. In truth, the symptoms are remarkably variable – one youngish patient, a Chinese martial arts trainer, was sure that something was wrong after a blow in the lower abdomen from one of her students, which she would normally have parried with ease, caused persistent pain for three weeks – and she was right. She had ovarian cancer and needed urgent surgery and chemotherapy. It is because of the vagueness of these symptoms that so many patients are finally diagnosed at a late stage. New methods of successful screening for ovarian cancer are badly needed (more on this later).

MOST COMMON SYMPTOMS OF OVARIAN CARCINOMA
Pelvic and/or abdominal mass 95%
Non-specific abdominal discomfort 75%
Abdominal bloating 55%
Early satiety 45%
Ascites 40%
Weight loss 30%
Shortness of breath 20%
Vaginal bleeding 10%
Urinary frequency 10%
Pleural effusion 10%

treatment

Patients with gynaecological cancer, or even the suspicion of it, need immediate referral to a specialist to confirm or exclude the diagnosis, by surgical biopsy in the case of accessible cancers – vulva, vagina, cervix – or by dilatation and curettage (D and C, or 'scraping') of the womb, in the case of cancer of the uterus. The dilatation refers to the simple stretching procedure to open up the cervix in order to introduce the proper instrument through the uterus into the womb, to take samples (curettings) for biopsy purposes. With ovarian cancer, pre-operative biopsy confirmation is not usually possible, but examination and scanning generally give a pretty fair indication of what the diagnosis is likely to be.

PRE-OPERATIVE ASSESSMENT

Before definitive surgery it is important to stage patients wherever possible to gain a detailed idea of the degree of spread in order to carry out the best possible treatment. Careful staging also allows the treatment results from one centre to be compared with those of another. Increasingly, staging will include CT or MRI scans, but also important is the examination under anaesthesia (EUA), which will allow the surgeon to inspect, see and feel for him- or herself the degree of local spread of the tumour without actually performing a surgical procedure on that occasion. With cancers of the vulva and cervix, this may well determine whether an operation is the best way forward, or whether the patient would be better treated with radiotherapy instead.

WHICH IS THE BEST TREATMENT?

All gynaecological cancers have the potential for spread, and surgery is only likely to be successful with relatively contained tumours – neither the patient nor the surgeon will be very satisfied if an operation is performed with the aim of cure, but the findings on the operating table prove more advanced than expected. Careful pre-operative assessment should cut down on this as far as possible.

● **For vulval and lower vaginal cancers**, the most common routes of spread are to local lymph nodes (generally those in the groin or more deeply within the pelvis).

● **Cancer of the cervix** tends to spread both locally, towards the pelvic side wall, and also upwards through lymph node spread. These features are not uncommon in cancer of the cervix, and if present, usually rule out surgery as a serious option.

● **With ovarian cancer**, the clinical behaviour is altogether different. These tumours spread widely, typically upwards to the abdominal cavity, sometimes with tumour deposits covering the internal lining of the abdomen, frequently producing tumour fluid, which can cause abdominal distension. If the tumour is well localised, surgery or radiotherapy for gynaecological cancer will offer an excellent chance of cure.

Common sites of secondary deposits (metastases) in ovarian cancer. This cancer has an unusual pattern of spread, largely within the pelvis and abdomen rather than more distantly as with so many types of cancer.

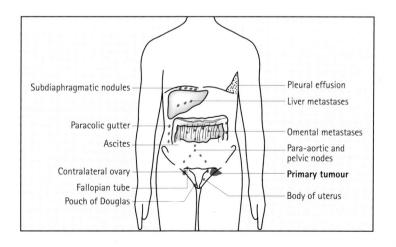

Subdiaphragmatic nodules

Paracolic gutter

Ascites

Contralateral ovary

Fallopian tube

Pouch of Douglas

Pleural effusion

Liver metastases

Omental metastases

Para-aortic and pelvic nodes

Primary tumour

Body of uterus

No one should underestimate the profound psychological trauma of gynaecological cancer surgery, and no surgeon would recommend a major operation, such as radical hysterectomy, without due thought. The aim, of course, is to eradicate the cancer without any need for additional treatment, such as radiotherapy. The operation is used for relatively localised invasive cancers of the cervix; with any degree of spread apart from minimal extension beyond the cervix itself, surgery is usually regarded as inappropriate since radiotherapy offers better results.

The results of radiotherapy for early tumours are as good as with surgery, but surgery is preferred in younger, fit women, because the side-effects tend to be less problematic. It is usually possible to preserve one or both ovaries surgically, thus retaining the normal hormonal profile, whereas with radiotherapy, pelvic irradiation always destroys ovarian function. Secondly, the dose of radiotherapy, may lead to significant late side-effects such as bowel damage or shrinkage of the bladder capacity. With more advanced cancers, or in patients who are too elderly, unfit, or unsuitable for surgery, there is no choice, radiotherapy offering the only chance of cure.

Most patients who have the right type of surgery for a localised cancer of the cervix, vulva or uterus are totally cured. In uterine cancer, post-operative treatment with radiotherapy, for those who need it, will cure many more. For surgically incurable patients, treatment of cancer of the cervix by radiotherapy can also be extremely successful, even curative, depending on the stage of disease. Very advanced cases are extremely difficult to cure by any means. Ovarian cancer is also curable in its early stages, but more advanced cases, with spread beyond the pelvis, are much more difficult to cure, though many patients live for years if responsive to chemotherapy. These are patients who would almost certainly not have survived beyond six months from diagnosis, so chemotherapy is most certainly justifiable, even if not always curative. With modern supportive care, including anti-nausea therapy, most patients get through the treatment without too much difficulty.

TREATMENT OF OVARIAN CANCER

Surgery: Surgical removal is extremely important, even in cases where the tumour has clearly spread beyond the ovary (sadly, the majority); a form of treatment which provides 'debulking' in a way that no other method can quite match. With locally advanced tumours it may be necessary for the surgeon to perform a lengthy procedure, to reduce tumour bulk to a level where chemotherapy can then be offered with a real chance of success. Surgical cure of ovarian cancer is certainly achievable in localised cases, but these form no more than 20%, at best.

Chemotherapy: This is of real value in the larger group with more extensive disease, particularly where surgical excision has been possible. It is now given routinely in ovarian cancer, including the more

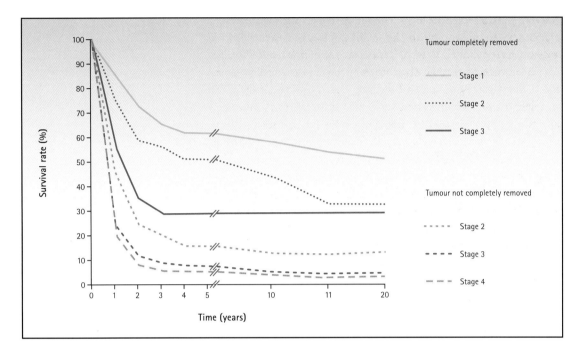

The graph demonstrates the importance of surgical removal of as much tumour tissue as possible in ovarian cancer.

Stage 1: tumour confined to the ovary itself.

Stage 2: tumour has extended to other pelvic sites.

Stage 3: tumour involves abdominal structures, i.e. it is well beyond the true pelvis.

Stage 4: the tumour is even more advanced.

advanced cases where the patient is fit enough to cope with it (fortunately, the majority). It generally lasts for about six months and is given as intermittent pulses of intravenous therapy (usually with combinations of drugs) every three or four weeks depending on the blood count, usually for a total of six courses. There is no definite evidence as to which is the best choice of agents, and many trials are in progress. One point of agreement is that either cisplatin or its more recent derivative, carboplatin, should be used. The other widely used chemo drug with considerable activity in ovarian cancer is Taxol (see page 213).

There is a very small but important group of ovarian tumours generally developing in younger patients and known as teratomas, or germ cell tumours, in which chemotherapy is usually curative. These are very similar in nature to the far more common testicular teratoma group, described on page 123. Although rare, if they are accurately diagnosed they are highly curable, when the appropriate chemotherapy is given.

Second-look laparotomy: Some patients with ovarian cancer are recommended to have a second-look laparotomy, an operation performed after completion of chemotherapy, to see what has been achieved. The need for a second-look laparotomy is really a recognition that scanning and other methods are not completely able to determine the true state of affairs. The value of this procedure does remain in doubt though, since some specialists argue that, if residual disease is confirmed, there is often little more to be done about it. Further chemotherapy may be valuable, at least in the short term, but there is no denying that the presence of residual disease after six courses of chemotherapy is obviously a bad sign, since long-term survivors are likely to come from the 'no residual disease' group. On the other hand, not all patients are able to undergo the ideal form of debulking surgery prior to chemotherapy; in a proportion, when chemotherapy has really begun to shrink the tumour masses, a second-look laparotomy can be justifiable to complete a reduction of bulky disease for the first time. Radiotherapy also has its place in ovarian cancer, but with only a limited role.

TREATMENT OF CERVICAL CANCER

Surgery: Radical hysterectomy is the treatment of choice for younger patients with localised disease. Most are cured, though permanent loss of fertility cannot be avoided. It is usually possible to conserve the ovaries, so hormonal and sexual function are better than with radiotherapy. Surgery cannot be undertaken with curative intent if the tumour has started to progress beyond the cervix. Very occasionally for exceptionally early invasive cancer in young women, a more conservative procedure (trachellectomy) can be considered, in which the cervix itself is surgically removed but the uterus is otherwise left intact. This highly controversial and relatively new approach may be a realistic alternative for women concerned about their future fertility.

Radiotherapy: This is often remarkably successful, even where surgical cure is clearly impossible by virtue of local progression of disease or lymph-node involvement. Treatment is likely to be by a combination of external and internal approaches, most centres in the UK preferring to use external radiation first, and then internal treatment, performed under spinal or general anaesthetic. In the last few years, several clinical trials have shown that routine use of chemotherapy together with radiation gives even better results than radiotherapy alone; chemoradiation has become the standard treatment for inoperable cases.

Unfortunately all approaches, whether principally surgical or by radiotherapy, carry a risk of both short- and long-term side-effects. For potentially fatal invasive cancer, there really is no other way than to accept a small risk as the possible price of cure. With surgery, the operation has to be radical to be adequate at all; with radiotherapy, the dose has to be high for the best chance of success. Although the risk of severe, late-onset side-effects from radiotherapy is not all that great, quite a number of patients do complain of more minor problems, such as persistent loose bowels or intermittent abdominal discomfort. The more severe symptoms result from radiation damage to the bowel, occasionally to the point where the affected area has to be removed.

TREATMENT OF UTERINE CANCER

Surgery: For uterine cancer, the good news is that most patients are curable by a relatively straightforward hysterectomy (of a less radical variety than for cancer of the cervix), together with removal of the ovaries (most patients are post-menopausal anyway, so this doesn't usually cause too much of a problem).

Radiotherapy: Patients with significant invasion of the muscular wall of the uterus or other adverse features are usually recommended to have post-operative radiotherapy, either with external methods or an intra-vaginal application, or sometimes with both to give additional protection against local recurrence.

prognosis

Careful follow-up is essential, ideally in a joint clinic where the gynaecologist and oncologist see the patient together. Skilled counselling can be extremely helpful – hardly surprising, in view of the particular problem posed by gynaecological cancers.

In the long term, many patients may well be cured, but with physical or emotional scars that can take years to heal, particularly in younger women, who may have to face not only a life-threatening illness, but also loss of fertility, sexuality and body image. In patients with cancer of the cervix, sex may become more difficult because of the surgical shortening of the vagina or the radiotherapy effect of vaginal dryness and atrophy (thinning of the vaginal lining) from hormonal loss after irradiation. HRT can be given safely and should be offered as a matter of course, at least in most patients. It helps to offset many problems but is not enough by itself. Counselling and reassurance will be needed long after the treatment has been completed. Few patients are able simply to 'snap back' into a normal family life when their own has been so disastrously disrupted.

There are some gynaecological cancers, however, in which HRT is ill-advised, notably cancer of the womb in which over-oestrogenisation may have been the cause. Glandular cancers of the cervix (adenocarcinoma), may also be hormone sensitive. In these patients, a newer form of non-oestrogen HRT (Livial) is less of a worry and can be extremely effective. HRT seems pretty safe in patients who have undergone treatment for ovarian cancer. Since excess oestrogen production is not regarded as a risk factor for ovarian cancer, there seems no logical reason to avoid it.

In summary, gynaecological cancers are a very mixed bag. Many are curable, but early diagnosis and treatment are the key. It's always tragic to encounter a patient who could have been cured early on, but wrong diagnosis, inadequate treatment or, occasionally, the patient's own disinclination to follow medical advice have made this impossible. One still sees the odd patient who follows the 'alternative' path, takes megadoses of vitamins and a highly excluding diet, and falls prey to an unskilled 'healer'. The last such patient coming through our department was even assured that these methods had led to complete healing of the cancer; no tests, of course – just the certainty of the ignorant. A couple of months later she turned up with obviously advancing disease, finally agreeing to an operation at a time when it was clearly too late. It breaks your heart.

BREAST CANCER

Breast cancer has reached almost epidemic proportions in the Western world, with well over 20,000 new cases occurring annually in England and Wales alone; one of the highest incidence rates in the world. In British women, breast cancer is by far the most common cancer of all, both in incidence and fatalities (about 20% of all female cancers). Media interest has never been higher, research into breast cancer has never been more active, yet progress has been slower than for some of the other types of cancer.

At least one in twelve Western women will develop the disease during their lifetime. Three-quarters will be in the postmenopausal period of life, i.e. over the age of 50, and it's in this group that mammographic screening appears to produce the greatest benefit. The principle, of course, is that small tumours, so small that they may be impossible to feel, can nonetheless be detected by mammography and therefore be more successfully treated than larger tumours with, at the end of the day, a better chance of survival. An important part of the rationale for screening in this group is that the disease is so common in the unselected female population that the pick-up rate will be high enough to justify both the expense and anxiety caused by the call back for further testing or biopsy in a woman who might turn out to have a benign breast disorder – also an extremely common diagnosis, far more so than breast cancer itself. To assess the real benefit of screening, it's not enough simply to state in a research publication that so many cases of cancer had been picked up and treated earlier than otherwise would have been possible; this observation does not in itself prove that the whole endeavour was necessarily worthwhile. We need to know that earlier treatment of screen-detected cancers really does lead to better survival. Research from the UK strongly suggests that the recommendation of a three-year interval between mammography screening tests will certainly fail to pick up substantial numbers of cases.

Almost all breast cancers arise from the glands lining the milk-forming ducts and their tributaries, in other words they are typical adenocarcinomas (see page 28). True invasive breast cancer is recognisable pathologically in a surgical biopsy specimen because the so-called basement membrane of the duct will have been breached as the tumour cells spill into the deeper tissues of the breast itself. Non-invasive, or intraduct, breast cancer is also well recognised, though the two conditions can co-exist. It can occur at several sites within the breast. Although the national recommendations for frequency and age group for screening are quite specific, there are clearly patients who ought to be examined mammographically more frequently, though it's difficult to be more specific. Patients with breast cancer are usually followed up with mammograms every 12 to 18 months. The higher the risk (see box, below), the more reasonable it seems to start screening at an earlier age. In a very extreme example, one might envisage a young woman of 35, with no children herself and a very strong family history of breast cancer, including an identical twin sister who, out of the blue, revealed that she had developed breast cancer three years beforehand, but had not told her twin for fear of upsetting her. Obviously a woman like this should be screened regularly at yearly intervals though in most women risk factors would obviously be far less dramatic than in the illustration above. Occasionally a woman in a very high risk group (such as the example given above) might be offered removal of all the breast tissue but with preservation of the skin and nipple, with immediate surgical reconstruction (see page 89). More and more surgeons feel that this kind of approach may have a place in highly selected patients.

causes

Quite a lot about the causation of breast cancer is now known:

● It's clearly a disease in which a family history is important, and women with a first-degree relative with breast cancer have a threefold increase in risk. The more relatives, the higher the risk, particularly where the relative developed the tumour herself at a young age.

● Women with no children, or who have their first pregnancy after the age of 30, are at about three times the risk of those who had their first pregnancy at 20 or younger.

● The risk also increases with a late menopause or early age when the periods first start.

● There's also quite a lot of evidence suggesting a link with our relatively high-fat diet, a feature of Western lifestyles, though the point is far from proven.

● Data from Hiroshima points quite clearly to radiation being a cause, though it took far longer to recognise breast cancer as being increased in incidence (about 35 years) than with other types of radiation-induced tumour also caused by the bomb, presumably a reflection of the unusually slow 'biological evolution' or tempo of breast cancer in its early stages of development.

● It has also been suggested that hormone replacement therapy (HRT), now so widely used, may be associated with a small increase in the risk of breast cancer. The latest figures are as follows: between ages 50 and 70 years (i.e. the most common period for a woman to take HRT), about 45 per 1,000 women not using HRT will be diagnosed. For those taking HRT for five years, two extra cases would be diagnosed per 1,000 women, by the age of 70. If you take HRT for ten years the figure rises by an extra six cases and for 15 years' use, by 12 extra cases. However, it also seems clear that the risk comes down – probably back to normal

FACTORS AFFECTING THE RISK OF DEVELOPING BREAST CANCER

Well-established
● Increasing age.
● Reproductive factors: early age at menarche, nulliparity, late age at first birth (more than 30 years), late age at menopause.
● Family history.
● Rare inherited familial syndromes.
● Previous history of breast cancer.
● Benign breast disease proven on biopsy.
● Ionising radiation.

Weakly associated or under evaluation
● Oral contraception, hormone replacement therapy.
● Dietary: obesity (post-menopausal women), high-fat diet.
● Alcohol.

Possible protective factors
● High levels of physical activity.
● Breast feeding.
● Diets high in fibre.
● High intake of fresh fruit and vegetables.

again – after five years' cessation of use. Interestingly, the size of the increased risk is virtually identical to what is seen with a naturally delayed or late menopause. What's more, patients on HRT are – as a group – more likely to have regular screening checks anyway, so it may well be a case of picking up a breast cancer earlier, rather than a genuine increase in the risk of developing the disease. And the benefits of HRT are, of course, considerable.

Patients with breast cancer often ask how long they have had it, and it's never really possible to say. All cancers are thought to begin with mutation of a single cell, well before any possibility of recognition by any known method. Some are genetically predetermined, probably by a particular gene sequence in affected individuals. Since it is known that it took 35 years for a slight but real statistical increase in the number of women developing breast cancer after the radiation blast at Hiroshima to show up, it is probably safe to assume that most breast cancers start their development many years (probably decades) before they make their visible or palpable appearance.

There are certainly wide differences in incidence across the world – high in Europe and North America, low in many parts of Asia and Africa. In Britain, the overall incidence is clearly rising, with the largest increase, 11%, noted in the decade between 1968 and 1978. This may well continue since, with changing social patterns, better obstetrics and more efficient methods of contraception, women are putting off the age of their first pregnancy until later and later. The mean age of first pregnancy is now 28 years – more than a decade beyond the age at which childbearing would otherwise normally begin.

symptoms and diagnosis

Apart from patients who present through screening programmes, the main symptomatic group – still the majority – usually come to their GPs with a lump in the breast which either they or their partner have felt. Most women know that the sooner they seek medical advice, the better. Some patients know their breasts intimately, some not; some have had so much trouble over the years with cysts, recurrent breast pain, benign breast problems of one type or another that they live in constant fear of developing breast cancer and bring any new finding to their doctor's attention without delay. The other, more laid back, type of patient may be just as liable, though, to develop the illness and by far the most sensible advice must be to show any breast lump to the doctor and let him or her decide what's to be done.

There is a ten to one chance that it is benign. This is a fairly consistent figure, but even an experienced surgeon may find it impossible to be certain of the nature of the lump, even after a thorough examination, without at the very least a mammogram (or ultrasound in younger women), possibly even a biopsy. Mammograms are pretty safe nowadays, with a far lower risk of radiation exposure than previously, and no

MOST COMMON SYMPTOMS OF BREAST CANCER
Lump 90% Painful lump 20% Nipple change 10% Nipple discharge 3% Skin contour change 5%

apparent danger, as far as one can tell, even when repeated on a regular basis every two years or so. This may seem inconsistent with the earlier story of the two sisters with breast cancer, but many believe that it is the timing which matters, the developing breast of a young teenage girl being far more sensitive from the carcinogenic (cancer risk) point of view than the mature breast – and anyway, a mammogram nowadays delivers less radiation than a chest X-ray.

HOW DOES A BREAST CANCER FEEL?

- Usually the lump is fairly firm, often situated quite close to the nipple and most typically in the upper outer quadrant of the breast rather than the lower part or the inner portion.
- Most breast cancers are painless but slightly tender when pressed or squeezed.
- Nipple discharge is unusual, unless the cancer actually involves the area just behind the nipple itself.
- The skin is generally normal in appearance, but a cancer situated close to the surface can distort it, producing a characteristically dimpled appearance, sometimes particularly evident when the patient leans forward and the breast hangs more freely.
- If there are obvious glands in the armpit, this is further evidence that the lump could well be malignant. The rest of the breast – away from the lump – and the other breast generally feel normal.
- If there is an ulcer, i.e. the surface of the skin is broken, this also is an important visible sign of possible cancer, and the same applies to an obvious elevation of the area of skin corresponding to the lump. Do not delay! See the doctor, then you will know.
- Patients with tender, painful breasts, particularly when the cycle of discomfort corresponds to the menstrual period, can almost always be reassured that the cause is benign. See also opposite.

Confirmation of the diagnosis is usually performed as an out-patient by the surgeon in the breast clinic, who will be the first port of call after referral from the family doctor. In the bad old days, patients were often subjected to what is now regarded as a pretty barbaric approach: 'We'll put you under an anaesthetic, remove the lump, and, if immediate examination confirms it's cancer, we'll perform a mastectomy there and then.' This approach has, thankfully, been pretty much abandoned now, and patients are usually treated with greater sensitivity and the diagnosis confirmed (or excluded) by fine-needle aspiration of the breast lump, performed as an out-patient. This involves a simple procedure where the surgeon (or sometimes an expert pathologist) inserts a fine needle and syringe combination, just as for breast cysts, sucking gently in order to produce a tiny volume of material, which can immediately be smeared on to a microscope slide. This simple technique (though it does take skill, and a certain knack, to get reliable results) provides plenty of cells spread out thinly, generally allowing diagnosis

SURVIVAL OF PATIENTS WITH BREAST CANCER ACCORDING TO INVOLVEMENT OF ARMPIT LYMPH NODES

Survival at 10 years
Negative armpit lymph nodes:
64.9%

Positive armpit lymph nodes: 24.9%

1-3 nodes involved:
37.5%

More than 4 nodes involved: 13.4%

BREAST AWARENESS

Being breast aware is an important part of caring for your body. This means knowing how your breasts look and feel so that if you should notice any change you will spot it early. If cancer should then be diagnosed, any treatment may well have a better outcome. If you are aged between 50 and 64 you are entitled to be screened every three years as part of the National Breast Screening Programme – you will be contacted via your GP's list. Breast screening is also available for women over 40 from private health-screening centres. Men too need to be aware of any changes in their breast tissue: about 200 men in the UK get breast cancer each year.

To help become familiar with your breasts
• Use a mirror in a good light so that you can *see* your breasts from different angles. First let your arms hang loosely by your sides and then raise them above your head. Turn from side to side.
• Then *feel* your breasts: you might find this easier with a soapy hand in the bath or shower or you might prefer to do it lying down.
• Use your right hand to examine your left breast and your left hand to examine your right. Put the hand you're not using behind or under your head. It helps to put a folded towel under your shoulder blade on the side you are examining as the breast tissue then spreads more readily.
• Use your fingers together and the flat of the fingers, not the tips. Start from the collarbone above your breast and trace a continuous spiral around your breast in small circles. Feel gently but firmly for any unusual lump or thickening. Finally, examine your armpit starting in the hollow and working down towards your breast.
• Ensure the timing is convenient and that you feel comfortable: the best time to do it is just after a period, when your breasts are usually softest and no longer tender. If you've stopped having periods, do it, say, on the first day of each month.
• Remember that there are always times when your breasts will feel different and for natural reasons. They are affected by hormonal changes during your menstrual cycle, pregnancy, breast feeding, the menopause and through weight loss and gain.

As you explore your breasts, be aware of the following points:
• a change in breast size - perhaps one breast becomes larger or lower.
• an inverted nipple or a nipple that has changed position or shape.
• a rash around the nipple.
• discharge from one or both nipples.
• puckering or dimpling of the skin.
• a swelling under your armpit or around your collarbone.
• a lump or thickening in your breast that feels different from the rest of the breast tissue.
• constant pain in one part of your breast or in your armpit.

What to do if you find a change
If you do find a change, no matter how small, go to see your GP. Don't worry that you might be making a fuss but also remember that many breast changes are benign and harmless. Your GP will want to examine your breasts and he or she may be able to reassure you that there is nothing to worry about. Alternatively, your GP may send you to a breast clinic for a more detailed examination.

of a malignant tumour or benign disorder to be made with complete confidence, though occasionally the test may have to be repeated if the initial result is equivocal.

treatment

If the aspiration test confirms cancer, the next step is to decide on the appropriate operation. Twenty years ago, this was a simple matter – patients were treated by mastectomy, the more radical the better. However, over the past 25 years there has been a complete rethink about this.

BREAST PRESERVATION
There is excellent evidence from several large studies that local excision (lumpectomy) together with post-operative radiotherapy generally gives results at least as good as mastectomy, though obviously there are exceptions. For the most part, the preserved breast looks excellent, has a normal nipple, with a natural feel to it and no loss of sensation. Usually, no surgical reconstruction will be necessary. For all these reasons, more and more surgeons are happy to restrict the surgical removal to a lumpectomy, generally combined with the removal of the glands from the armpit area (axilla). This achieves both surgical control and provides the best possible information about the presence or absence of lymph node involvement from the tumour. This is extremely important,

ESTABLISHING WHETHER THE CANCER HAS SPREAD

Initial staging procedures in patients with breast cancer can be kept very limited. Some years ago there was a vogue for performing a whole series of procedures including abdominal ultrasound examination, isotope bone scanning and a wide variety of blood tests in all cases; it is now known that the pick-up rate of these investigations is extremely low – indeed, some patients suffer considerable unnecessary anxiety since the tests can give a 'false positive' picture. Although breast cancer cells can, of course, spread at a microscopic level to the axillary (and neck) lymph nodes and, even more important, via the bloodstream to distant parts of the body (bone, liver, lung, brain and so on), these potential metastatic sites cannot usually be recognised by the current scanning or blood-testing techniques, again arguing in favour of avoiding them altogether.

Better ways of establishing whether patients do have secondary spread are urgently needed; a reliable tumour marker would obviously be best, but at the moment no reliable ones have emerged. The best guide to future events is the presence and degree of lymph node involvement of the axilla, with a strong body of evidence that it gives a quantitative estimate of outcome. For example, those with ten or more positive lymph nodes clearly do worse, as a group, than those with, say, five nodes, who in turn have a less satisfactory prognosis than those with only one or two. In some centres, a more restricted node-examining procedure is carried out ('sentinel-node' biopsy), though it is still best regarded as a research tool. In this test, use of a radioactive dye (injected directly into the breast, close to the cancer) outlines the first, or sentinel, node to which the cancer might spread. This is then removed and examined, and the result seems to correlate closely with the more formal axillary dissection.

since this feature provides the clearest indicator as to the likely out-come (see box, page 88).

Patients with small primary tumours, for example, and no evidence of involvement in a good sample of ten or more axillary lymph nodes have a good outcome, and are quite difficult to distinguish statistically from the normal population, at least for the first ten years after diagnosis and treatment. On the other hand, in a young woman with a large primary tumour and heavy axillary lymph node involvement, the outcome is much less satisfactory and further treatment with chemotherapy, hormone therapy or both will be necessary (more about this on pages 93-6).

MASTECTOMY

Some patients are, however, better treated by mastectomy than breast preservation. First of all, there are patients with relatively large but still operable tumours in a small breast, in whom an attempt at lumpectomy would produce a very misshapen and cosmetically unsatisfactory result. Far better to do a simple mastectomy, possibly with primary breast reconstruction or – to many patients' satisfaction – the use of an external prosthesis. Second, there are certain patients who prefer to undergo mastectomy, feeling rightly or wrongly that they would sooner go the whole hog in order to be as safe as possible. It would be quite wrong to bully these patients away from a firmly held view, even if technically the lumpectomy procedure were possible. Finally, patients with a centrally placed tumour, just behind the nipple, may sometimes be better off with a mastectomy since local excision would require removal of the nipple, a serious cosmetic, sexual and emotional loss, though this is very much a matter for discussion between the surgeon and the patient (and perhaps the patient's partner as well, if she wishes).

It is well worth remembering that for all the advantages of a preserved breast, the necessary post-operative radiotherapy can be arduous and never accomplished as quickly as a mastectomy, so elderly or frail patients may be better treated by mastectomy, if they do not object to the operation. This will spare them the inconvenience of radiotherapy, particularly if they happen to live far from an oncology centre and don't have a strong preference for breast-preserving treatment. Needless to say, not all patients have the same priorities when it comes to sense of body image, concerns about intimacy and sexuality, etc.

RADIOTHERAPY

The risk of local recurrence following lumpectomy alone is so high – at least 35% – that radiotherapy is almost always recommended, even though, admittedly, a local recurrence within the breast is not usually a life-threatening event. However, any recurrent event in breast cancer is best avoided, and most specialists endorse this general view; and there is evidence that a local recurrence may to some extent predict for a

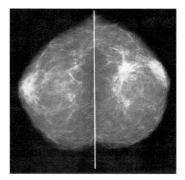

Some breast cancers – though not all – are obvious on the mammogram, as in this case where the tumour is clearly visible. The images show the left and right breasts (side view). The left breast is normal (on the left side). A cancer is clearly visible deep within the substance of the right breast.

RADIOTHERAPY AND BREAST CANCER

In the short term, patients can expect to remain pretty well throughout the treatment, though most will experience a slight reddening of skin and/or discomfort in the treated area. The skin colour change may be more pronounced in pale-skinned patients and the outermost layer of skin may even partially peel off (dry desquamation). More serious skin damage (moist desquamation) is quite unusual these days, except in patients with large, pendulous breasts, where it may be difficult to avoid because of the apposition of skin surfaces at the under-surface of the breast. Where the dose is high, it can also occur in the axilla (armpit). In any event, these changes should be pretty short lived. The other treatment complications are relatively minor but worth mentioning – many patients feel tired and need to be reassured that this is normal, particularly in the latter half of treatment. Some may feel nauseated, especially at the start of treatment, though this settles down rapidly and is not generally a problem.

If you are undergoing a course of radiotherapy and want to carry on working, then do so since it can help sustain a sense of self-esteem, and avoids too much undesirable focusing on the illness at a time when the goal must surely be to get on and complete the treatment with as little upset and interruption as possible. The alternative to continuing with work is often an undesirable loss of self-confidence, and all too frequently one sees a disconsolate patient who feels that they are doing the right thing by 'resting', but becomes bored, irritable and anxious. It all depends on the individual, of course – some welcome an opportunity to take time off, particularly where the work is stressful and can't easily be performed in a half-hearted way. The ideal is usually to go in for, say, the morning and then leave early, coming into the department for treatment on the way home. This kind of detail is actually quite important since it helps patients retain a sense of control, a key feature in coming to terms with a threatening illness which only a month or two beforehand had not even been detected.

Some patients undergoing radiotherapy are advised not to wash the affected area during treatment because any skin reactions can sometimes be made worse, possibly due to the friction and force of towel drying. Individual skin reactions do vary considerably from patient to patient and the radiographer will give advice. In any event, patients will be seen and reviewed by one of the medical and nursing team on a regular weekly basis (more often, if necessary) so that important details such as skin reaction can be discussed and, if necessary, treated – generally with low-strength hydrocortisone cream, which usually works very well, though aloe vera and other non-steroidal applications are increasingly popular.

Most skin reactions settle very quickly, and after completion of the radiotherapy, patients will routinely be seen in clinic every three months or so for further review and examination. It's sensible for the mammogram to be repeated every 12 to 18 months, to keep a close watch on the other breast as well as to check on the one that has been irradiated.

more generalised recurrence, which of course is a far more significant and serious event.

There is no firm agreement on the specifics of the post-operative radiotherapy, some centres preferring a relatively short course, in the region of three weeks, while others go more slowly, taking the treatment over six weeks and with a lower radiation dose per day. Some regard this as an appalling and unjustifiable medical failing, arguing forcefully that the approach should be far more consistent as not everyone can be doing it right! On the other hand, this type of difference (in technical detail) is typical of many situations in medicine, where specialists offer an approach likely to be coloured by all sorts of influences, including their own training, philosophy and the resources available. Although some patients treated by radiotherapy for breast cancer do develop side-effects at a later stage (those with serious problems are fortunately a very tiny proportion of the numbers that are treated), there doesn't seem to be any clear evidence that, say, patients undergoing a rapid, three-week treatment course have more to fear from long-term side-effects than those who are treated at a slower rate over six weeks.

Patients undergoing lumpectomy or mastectomy don't usually have to stay in hospital long – a few days, if that, in the case of lumpectomy; a week, or sometimes less, for mastectomy. In most centres, patients are routinely offered information and support by a breast care nurse specialist at the time of diagnosis or shortly afterwards, and are likely to meet the radiation oncologist shortly after discharge from hospital, if they haven't already done so. Before radiotherapy starts, the patient's treatment has to be planned with particular care since all breasts are different and the anatomy of the surrounding area is complex, with many sensitive structures nearby.

Patients will usually attend just one radiotherapy planning session, at which all the measurements are taken by radiographers, usually with an outline of their breast as well, so that the measurements, physics, calculations and computing required for definition of the radiation field can be completed quickly, with the treatment itself commencing just a few days later. Generally, but not always, patients are recommended to have daily treatment, five days a week, for three to six weeks, depending on the local preferences in the centre they are attending. The treatment volume will always include the whole of the breast, but when a full axillary lymph node dissection has been performed surgically, there is no need to irradiate the armpit area at all; in fact, there are good reasons to stay away from it, since long-term swelling of the arm, from excess tissue fluid (lymphoedema) is likely to result from overtreatment of this area.

ADJUVANT DRUG TREATMENTS

Apart from the revolution in local treatment, which has led so rapidly to rejection of mastectomy as the 'gold standard', an equally dramatic series of developments has led to the majority of patients now being treated with prophylactic or adjuvant systemic therapy – drug treatment, either with chemotherapy, hormone therapy or both – in an attempt to forestall the development of life-threatening metastases. As mentioned earlier, many patients with breast cancer harbour 'micrometastases', microscopic deposits that cannot be visualised, but are present at the outset of the disease and not, of course, amenable to any form of local therapy, be it surgery or radiation.

SIDE-EFFECTS OF TAMOXIFEN

Side-effects are few, but can include hot flushes, weight gain, occasional nausea, vaginal bleeding or discharge (usually very mild, but sometimes worrying for the patient – both of these symptoms generally settle down), and symptoms resulting from the oestrogen blockade, such as changes to the hair, skin or nails. Tamoxifen is not a contraceptive, and pre-menopausal patients on tamoxifen should be regarded as potentially fertile, even though in some brands of the drug, the package insert claims that periods do stop. In our experience, they generally don't, though there may be a real benefit for patients who, for much of their lives, may have suffered from irregular periods, as they often discover that with tamoxifen, their periods are more or less normal – a real bonus. In the long term, there is certainly a very small risk of a tamoxifen-related increase in the incidence of uterine cancer, presumably because tamoxifen's complex action includes some pro-oestrogenic as well as anti-oestrogenic effects (so much so that tamoxifen is sometimes used in infertility clinics!); again, this side-effect is extremely unusual and does not begin to compare as a potential disadvantage with the life-saving properties of the drug in patients with breast cancer. Fortunately, most uterine cancers caused by tamoxifen use (and again it's important to stress how rare these are) would be picked up early and are highly curable by hysterectomy.

Tamoxifen: It became clear over ten years ago that the routine use of tamoxifen, a simple tablet preparation, could protect post-menopausal patients (i.e. 75% of all cases), not to anything like a complete degree but sufficient to justify this treatment as an essential part of management in this age group. Tamoxifen is a well-tolerated oral agent, developed in the UK and now used world-wide, which is chiefly effective because of its anti-oestrogenic properties, i.e. by depriving residual breast cancer cells of the essential oestrogen needed for continued growth. Tamoxifen is also valuable in pre-menopausal patients as well, and many use it routinely for all patients with oestrogen receptor positive [ER+ve] patients. The ER status is defined by a simple slide test on the original biopsy – ER+ve patients have receptors on the cell surface, which seem to 'lock on' to circulating oestrogen (the female hormone). These cells require the oestrogen for their continued growth, so use of tamoxifen or other anti-oestrogens starve the ER+ve breast cancer cell of its essential hormonal stimulus. For post-menopausal patients in particular, the benefits of tamoxifen are so clear that no patient should be denied the potential benefit unless they are among the very small group who find tamoxifen impossible to cope with, or are definitely ER–ve. One important and still unanswered question is just how long the tamoxifen should be given for. At the time of writing, five years is the usual recommendation.

Other hormone therapies: There are also alternative forms of these therapies, notably the use of a radiation or surgically induced menopause, which again has a solid weight of evidence to support it. For the most part, these treatments are less widely used and should be restricted to ER+ve pre-menopausal patients – many of whom will experience a treatment-induced menopause from chemotherapy anyway.

Chemotherapy: Like tamoxifen, chemotherapy has now been used for more than 20 years. The weight of evidence is now very strongly in favour of chemotherapy as standard adjuvant treatment for all pre-menopausal patients with lymph node positive disease, a group in which it clearly improves survival. There is also evidence that even in the node negative group (who do much better anyway), there is an increase in what is termed 'disease-free survival', i.e. the probability of a patient remaining clear of recurrent disease, either at the original site or elsewhere, during the follow-up period.

It may seem self-evident that any length-ening of disease-free survival should automatically translate into an improvement in the more important, life-or-death, overall survival figure, but in fact this is still far from clear – because of the relative effectiveness of some of the available treatments for patients with recurrent disease. It's an important point because on the one hand, there is a natural tendency to use chemotherapy (or any other potentially use-ful treatment) for all patients who might reasonably benefit, but on the other, would it be right and proper to give intensive treat-ment of this kind to patients who might remain free of disease a little longer, but in whom, ultimately, the overall survival figures are probably no different? Life would be much easier, of course, if the treatment were both straightforward, inexpensive and very easy to tolerate. Although tamoxifen more or less satisfies these criteria, the same claims cannot be made for chemotherapy.

Most pre-menopausal patients under the age of 50 and with node positive disease are now routinely offered chemotherapy, usually with six courses of a standard drug regimen known as CMF (like most chemo protocols, the name is an acronym of the component drugs, in this case cyclophosphamide, methotrexate, and fluorouracil), which has been in common use for about 20 years now and was initially pioneered by Italian and American oncologists. With modern anti-nausea drugs,

GWEN'S STORY

Gwen was 37 when she first went to an oncological specialist. A painter with a lengthy history of profound psychological disturbance, Gwen had made several serious suicide attempts. She was divorced, had no children, was introspective and emotionally unstable. She'd been well aware of a substantial lump in her breast for at least six months before finally going to see her GP, ostensibly with the quite unrelated problem of sleepless-ness and daily fatigue. It was only as she was about to leave that she mentioned the lump.

It was enormous, occupying almost all of her left breast. Although it hadn't ulcerated yet, it wouldn't have been more than a couple of weeks before this would have happened. The specialist who saw her the following day couldn't feel any glands under the arm and, surpris-ingly, the operation proved straightforward. Gwen declined both radiotherapy and chemotherapy, but was persuaded to take tamoxifen and to see her specialist regularly for follow-up treatment.

That was seven years ago. Since that time, she has never missed one of her appointments, hasn't looked back and psychologically seems healthier than before. She obviously enjoys confounding the statistics, but she knows perfectly well that, with breast cancer, you can never be quite sure.

It's interesting how many patients like Gwen do seem to find a new focus in their lives when faced with a truly desperate, potentially life-threatening illness.

this chemotherapy is generally well tolerated, almost invariably given on an out-patient basis and at approximately three- to four-week intervals, i.e. over a total period of just under six months, provided that the blood count remains satisfactory throughout. Side-effects are described on pages 48-52.

Although CMF is very well researched and its effects understood in considerable depth, oncologists are constantly on the lookout for superior treatments that might yield better results, particularly in groups of patients at higher risk of recurrence – such as those with a very large number of positive axillary lymph nodes in the operative specimen. As a result, more powerful agents might well be recommended right from the start, possibly as part of a clinical trial. It might be, for example, that the researchers are interested in a possible advantage in giving the drugs on a continuous, infusional basis – rather than the traditional, intermittent pulse approach with chemotherapy. At present, though, despite encouraging reports from the USA and elsewhere, it is far from proven that more intensive chemotherapy than CMF has definite superiority, at least in the majority of patients without especially adverse risk features such as heavy axillary node involvement.

Chemotherapy combined with bone marrow transplantation: One much-heralded approach is the use of very high-dose chemotherapy supplemented by autologous bone marrow transplantation or peripheral stem cell transfusion (see page 57) for high-risk breast cancer patients, a treatment pioneered by Professor Bill Peters in North Carolina (USA).

Unfortunately, the results seem less impressive in the longer term than seemed likely five years ago, when it was looking so encouraging. Other more successful approaches have used more powerful chemotherapy either prior to surgery or as a post-operative adjuvant programme. To clarify this and many other issues, randomised trials will provide the most reliable answer.

TREATMENT FOR RECURRENT DISEASE

Sadly, some patients with breast cancer do develop recurrent disease, either at the primary site or as a result of distant spread, for example in bone sites such as the spine, ribs, pelvis or thigh bone, or the lung, skin or brain. Obviously, the clinical features will vary widely, depending on the precise site and degree of involvement; it is impossible to list here the ways in which such secondary spread might become apparent, though these have been

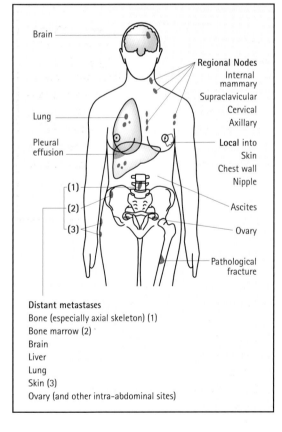

Brain

Regional Nodes
Internal mammary
Supraclavicular
Cervical
Axillary

Lung

Local into
Skin
Chest wall
Nipple

Pleural effusion

(1)
(2)
(3)

Ascites

Ovary

Pathological fracture

Distant metastases
Bone (especially axial skeleton) (1)
Bone marrow (2)
Brain
Liver
Lung
Skin (3)
Ovary (and other intra-abdominal sites)

Local, nodal and distant spread in breast cancer.

CHEMOTHERAPY AND BREAST CANCER

Some patients, probably the majority, will find that their menstrual cycle is substantially disrupted by chemotherapy, often to the point of complete cessation of periods. The closer the patient is to her expected menopause, the more likely this is to occur. Younger women given chemotherapy should be warned that it does not act as a contraceptive, nor is it likely to completely abolish the periods, even though they might be disrupted during the treatment itself. In young women, fertility is likely to be preserved and there are many instances of patients becoming pregnant afterwards. There's no guarantee, of course, so referral to an assisted-conception specialist is becoming more widely practised as egg storage (like sperm storage, which is now fully established) is fast becoming a reality. The question of whether or not the induction of a 'chemical' menopause of this kind is truly beneficial remains one of the uncertainties in this whole area, but many specialists believe that chemotherapy chiefly works via its effect on the ovary, so that if the patient continues to menstruate after six months' chemotherapy, the treatment should be augmented by pelvic irradiation or surgical removal of the ovaries, at least in ER+ve patients.

The trouble with the induction of the menopause at an early age is that it can produce sudden and very undesirable symptomatic side-effects – troublesome, persistent hot flushes, loss of libido, a tendency towards earlier osteoporosis and, sometimes, a whole cluster of symptoms related to chronological ageing, which some patients find hard to cope with. But to some extent, these can be prevented by the use of low-dose progesterone administration, which seems to work well with the majority of patients (though not all) and which seems completely safe. There is even an increasing view, contrary to traditional teaching, that hormone replacement therapy (HRT) is not unreasonable in selected patients who are greatly upset by the onset of this menopause. It may seem illogical to first produce a menopause deliberately and then offer hormone replacement, but in truth it's by no means illogical, since, for example, symptomatic HRT benefits can occur even though the dose of HRT, given in tablet or patch form, is substantially lower than the level of circulating oestrogens, which have been medically lowered. Once again, views on this difficult issue are divided, it may be safest to avoid routine HRT if it simply isn't necessary, but to use either progesterones or conventional HRT in selected symptomatic patients who requested it, or for patients with a strong family history of osteoporosis, which could represent a real threat to future health. There is no doubt that quality of life is in many respects much improved by the administration of HRT, a key issue in the decision-making process.

discussed to some extent on page 88. As far as treatment is concerned, the important thing, of course, is to weigh up the pros and cons of the various options with great care, and only use the treatments likely to be symptomatically beneficial. For instance, in a patient with a severe and localised discomfort as a result of a secondary deposit in a rib, a single dose of radiotherapy to the painful site will often produce excellent pain relief with little, if anything, in the way of troublesome side-effects. In general, radiotherapy offers an excellent chance of local pain control with bone secondaries at any site. A surgical stabilisation (internal orthopaedic fixation of a long bone, such as the femur for example) may also be useful in conjunction with radiotherapy. On the other hand, radiotherapy is difficult to use for abdominal secondary deposits, such as those arising within the liver, because of the limited tolerance of this

JACKIE'S STORY

Jackie, aged 52, from north London, has been married to Jim for 29 years and has two grown-up daughters.

There was a history of breast cancer in Jackie's side of the family – her mother had had breast cancer and also her great-grandmother so she has had a routine mammogram every two years. When it was time for her most recent mammogram, it had been two and a half years since she last had it so her GP arranged for it to be performed. After the mammogram, Jackie was asked to come back to the hospital in two days' time for a biopsy to be performed of a suspicious area in her breast. This was a shock for Jackie

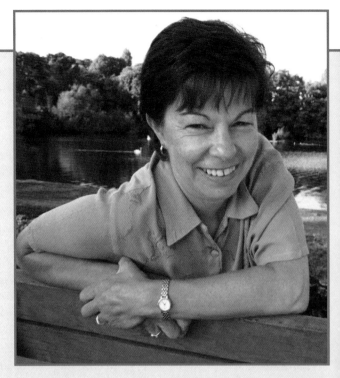

to realise something was wrong and that she may have breast cancer. The following week Jackie received the news in the out-patient clinic from the breast surgeon that the histological results from the tissue taken by the biopsy showed she had breast cancer and the recommended treatment was explained. Jackie was then seen by the breast care nurse specialist who explained again the options of treatment. Jackie's first thought at this time was 'just take it all away', she'd like a mastectomy, but by the following day she had changed her mind and had decided to have reconstruction surgery. Jackie had discussed the options available to her with her family and with her mother, who was now aged 83 and had had a bilateral mastectomy at the age of 53 – a year older than when Jackie had been diagnosed with breast cancer. Her mother had said, 'I still don't like looking at myself. If I had my chance again I'd definitely have reconstruction.'

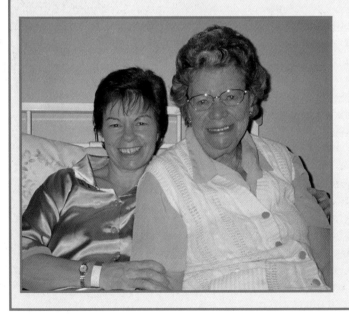

Not all breast tumours are suitable for conservative surgery such as breast reconstruction. Breast reconstruction may be performed at the time of the original mastectomy or later on. Jackie chose to have the former, avoiding having to have a second operation at a later date. Jackie recalls, 'My Mother was not told anything before her operation 30 years ago – but I was told everything. I was shown photos of what my breast would look like after the operation. You know I am not being funny but I don't feel like I have had my breast off.'

Jackie found the most difficult

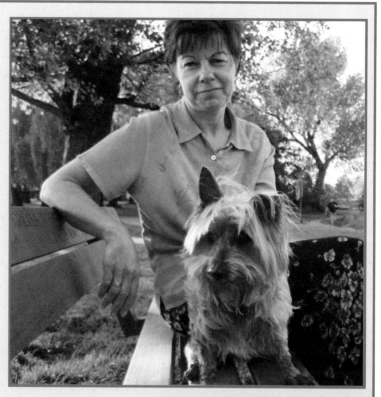

time was the wait of about five weeks for the operation to take place. She continued to go to work but found it difficult to concentrate at this time. Her main support came from her close family and many friends. For information she read CancerBACUP booklets and found these so helpful, especially in helping her to speak to family and friends, that she felt sufficiently well informed that she didn't feel the need to go to search the Internet.

Jackie has noticed how things have progressed for the better over the years. She had been 19 years old when her mother was diagnosed with cancer and 'cancer was not a thing you spoke about then.' Jackie's great grandmother had died of breast cancer but had not known that she had cancer as it was not mentioned. Jackie feels she is fortunate in that she did not require radiotherapy or chemotherapy treatment as well as the breast surgery. Jackie is also now going to arrange for her daughters to be seen in the Breast Family History Clinic. 'I think it is great there is now this programme and they can be checked.'

Jackie is grateful she had the routine mammogram as she said that in her case there was nothing to see and nothing to feel in her breast but the mammogram showed a suspicious area that needed to be further investigated. As Jackie says, 50% of women she had met in the hospital ward who had breast cancer had said the same. She is very positive for the future and admits that having a mother who has survived breast cancer has helped her enormously and says that if in the future she had to go through this treatment again she would. 'The surgeon says I can have more plastic surgery but I don't think I need more. I think it is great.'

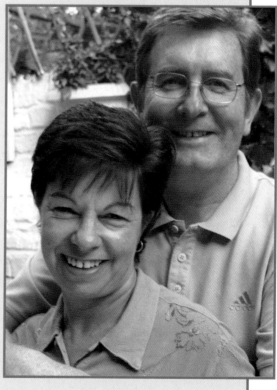

organ and the close proximity of other very sensitive structures. In these circumstances, chemotherapy is more likely to be helpful even in patients who have received previous adjuvant chemotherapy. If radiotherapy is the cornerstone of the treatment for bone and brain secondaries, chemotherapy (or possibly a change of hormone therapy, especially in patients known to be hormone responsive) is, on the whole, a better choice for lung, liver and/or glandular secondary deposits.

Even though patients with distant secondary spread are generally regarded as no longer curable, those with advanced or recurrent disease do quite often respond to alterations in their hormonal medication, and there is a wide variety of agents available. Most patients will have had treatment with tamoxifen as part of the initial or primary management; while some will have discontinued this treatment at the time of their relapse, others develop progressive disease while still taking it. For the first of these groups, particularly where they have been off the tamoxifen for several years beforehand, it makes sense to restart treatment with tamoxifen, since there may be an additional response. If, on the other hand, the relapse has occurred while the patient is actually taking it, there is little point in continuing with it, or at least relying on it as the sole treatment. The advice is usually to switch to a second-line hormone such as anastrazole (Arimidex), a potent anti-oestrogen that reduces the circulating oestrogen level to virtually unrecordable levels, or to use progesterone (typically given in much higher dosage than that which is used for symptomatic treatment of hot flushes). Although these drugs can be given by mouth, there are one or two other choices, which are typically given by monthly injections.

prognosis

Much has been written about the outlook or prognosis in breast cancer patients. Certainly it is one of the more unpredictable tumours, in the sense that patients who are free of disease, apparently cured, at five years after treatment, are not quite in the same position as those with, say, lung or testis cancer, where after five years free of recurrence, patients are almost certainly out of the woods. With breast cancer, it's rather different, since the disease can return at a later stage. This may be tough and unwelcome news, but although breast cancer is unusual in this regard, most of the relapses that occur do so within the first five years – some comfort, at least. It's also true that, on the whole, the later the disease recurs, the more likely the patient is to respond effectively to additional treatment when required – as if the tempo of the disease has a considerable bearing not only on its virulence, but also on the final outcome.

It was the recognition that breast cancer can return many years after it is first diagnosed and treated, at a distant site from the initial tumour, that led so many experts to begin to question the key importance of mastectomy in the first place. It took far too many decades and unnecessary operations for the medical profession to recognise that the real problem in breast cancer was not so much related to problems of local control, but rather the late, distant recurrence, which might eventually prove fatal.

Certainly in terms of prognosis, the smaller the tumour, the more likely the patient is to be cured by the initial treatment. As previously mentioned, other important pointers are:

● The lymph node status (whether positive or negative) as determined by the surgical dissection of the axillary nodes (generally regarded as the most important prognostic feature of all).

● The pathological 'grade' of the tumour, i.e. the degree of visible abnormalities in the cancer cells when viewed under the microscope. Some look very similar to normal breast tissue, others very bizarre.

The huge world-wide epidemic of breast cancer, so marked in the industrialised Western nations, has led to an explosion of research work. Although many are gloomy about the slow rate of change, the past 15 years or so have seen at least two major advances with real benefits for many patients: the confirmation that mastectomy is often quite unnecessary, replaced by far less damaging operations; and secondly, the confirmation that systemic agents such as tamoxifen and chemotherapy are clearly able to reduce recurrence and death rates. It's hard to predict what the next decade may bring, but certainly there are reasons to be cautiously optimistic about future progress.

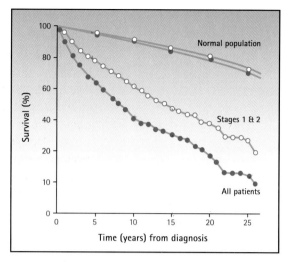

Survival rates for patients with breast cancer.

Stage 1: disease confined to the breast.

Stage 2: disease has spread to the axillary (armpit) lymph nodes.

All patients: this includes patients who may have had evidence of disease when first diagnosed. Over the past ten years, newer types of treatment have led to a significant improvement in these results.

GASTRO-INTESTINAL CANCER

The human gastro-intestinal tract is a remarkable and convoluted passageway between mouth and anus, capable of digesting an astonishing variety of foods, both nutritious and otherwise, turning even the most unlikely of substances into a valuable source of energy. Its various components have highly specialised functions; some are compact, such as the mouth and the gall bladder, whereas other parts, especially the small intestine, are lengthy and only contained within the body by ingenious feats of packaging. Although essentially tubular in nature, there are specialised glandular areas, such as the salivary glands, liver and pancreas, whose function is largely to manufacture and squirt in the appropriate enzymes at differing levels within the pathway, to assist the breakdown of foods into energy sources for the body.

Each of these sites can give rise to cancer, though, oddly enough, the small intestine, the longest by far, very rarely does so. In Western society, the most common sites for cancer are the mouth (see page 138), stomach and large bowel (though not necessarily in that order), although in other parts of the world, primary tumours of the liver or oesophagus are much more common. On the following pages we start at the top of the body and work down, beginning with the oesophagus (page 104) and then moving on to the stomach (page 105), the liver (page 107), the pancreas (page 108) and the bowel (page 110).

NIKKI'S STORY

Nikki is a 31-year-old who lives in north London and now works in IT. In January 1998, she noticed that one of her nipples was itchy; she had some shooting pains in the breast but she couldn't detect a lump. Two weeks later, however, she did find a lump and went to her GP who thought it might be an infection and so prescribed antibiotics. The antibiotics did not help so an ultrasound was performed, immediately followed by a mammogram. Nikki was accompanied by her boyfriend Craig and they were relieved that all the investigations were done so quickly.

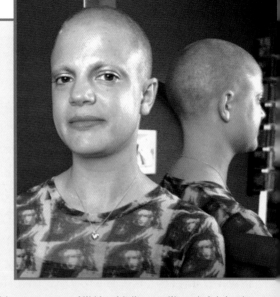

Nikki was seen by the breast surgeon who informed her that he would like to take a biopsy of the breast tissue for confirmation but that it did look as if she had breast cancer. Nikki said, 'It was like a brick in the face, it was like, right, OK, fine. But he was so honest and so up front and I really appreciated that because one of the biggest things I've found is that as a patient you need to make informed decisions. Every single decision I make has to be fully, fully informed and then I won't have any regrets about things that I have done or haven't done.' The biopsy was performed and cancer was confirmed. 'I went back to the surgeon and said how are you going to do the surgery and what are you going to do to keep the shape of the breast?' Nikki went ahead with the breast surgery. Both Craig and she found that they didn't get either really upset or really down. They just got on with it.

Then Nikki had to undergo further tests before being given high dose chemotherapy. At this time she and Craig had to consider the issue of fertility as the high dose chemotherapy would render Nikki infertile. They were referred to the fertility clinic for advice and possible options. Soon afterwards, a bone scan detected an abnormality and a tissue biopsy confirmed that it was a bone metastasis in the sternum. Nikki found this result devastating as she had discussed earlier the possibility that if the cancer had spread to the bones the disease was likely to be incurable.

However, it was decided that as Nikki was young and fit she should begin on the first part of a

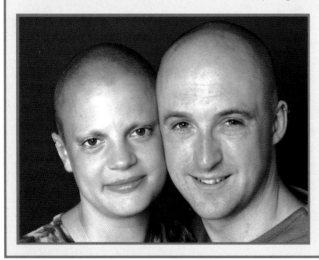

chemotherapy protocol, which consisted of three months of out-patient chemotherapy. If there was a response to the chemotherapy then the oncologists would proceed to a high dose chemotherapy treatment. There was a response, so the high dose treatment went ahead with Nikki spending three weeks in hospital.

Once the chemotherapy was completed, Nikki underwent six weeks of radiotherapy treatment. During this time she went back to her work as a nurse on the Intensive Care Unit and also to university where she was studying for a Performing Arts degree.

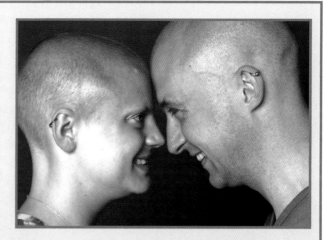

However, some months later the metastasis just above the sternum required some treatment, so a further six weeks of radiotherapy treatment was given. Nikki fitted this around her work at the hospital. Then she found that she was getting pain in her back, which she put down to the strain of nursing again and it wasn't until she was in tears with the pain that she went to her doctor. 'I didn't want to know that the cancer had spread. That was the one thing I was terrified of. I went as far as going to an osteopath rather than go to the hospital because I didn't want to know. Eventually I went back to the hospital and an ultrasound was performed. Spinal metastases were diagnosed and that was the turning point. I needed to know what the prognosis was. I didn't expect them to say three years. I regretted asking it – but more for the effect it had on us. But I still had to know and now I'm glad I know.'

Nikki says it was hard for herself, Craig and her family. This all changed the way they had thought about their lives – at the age of 27 – things like marriage and children. It was during this difficult time that Nikki and Craig decided to get married – they had been together since they were sixteen. Even though she had begun another course of chemotherapy, they were married in Las Vegas by an Elvis Presley look-alike and had a huge party in Scotland for family and friends once they had returned home. The chemotherapy dose was reduced while she was away and then, after all the wedding celebrations, Nikki completed the course with the dose back on a higher level. Although Nikki has lost her hair through chemotherapy treatment several times, she never wears a wig. 'I wear my baldness proudly, as a fashion statement. I make it fun with henna tattoos, which makes me feel more comfortable about myself and fits in well with my lifestyle.'

Nikki has found that complementary therapies have helped her enormously, especially yoga. 'Yoga is a time for me. It helps me to completely relax. I concentrate on trying to heal myself through visualisation and statements about what I want.' She has found that it strengthens her body and loosens her joints, especially her back. 'I get a huge amount of benefit from this and feel very positive afterwards.'

When asked how she has coped with her illness Nikki says, 'Work keeps me busy, it gives me a chance to socialise and funds trips and my social life, which are important to me. Also, having a positive attitude I always find that no matter how bad things get, there is usually something positive either in it or as a result of it. I try to live my life as normally as possible and NOT through cancer.'

Of her goals, Nikki says, 'Having a disease like this makes you determined to do all the things you have wanted to do but never got around to. I now keep planning nights out, weekends away and holidays so that I have goals to aim for and things to look forward to. I have a list of things to do in life and I am determined to do everything on it! One of them is to swim with dolphins.'

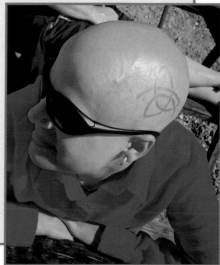

OESOPHAGEAL CANCER

Cancer of the oesophagus, or gullet, is more common in men (about two-thirds of all cases), with a peak incidence between 60 and 80 years. It has increased dramatically in incidence in the UK over the past decade, probably due to a dietary cause (though it is not quite known what is responsible). There is a very wide variation in incidence in different parts of the world. In the southern tip of South Africa, for example, it is one of the most common cancers; the same is true in parts of Russia and northern China. In the upper part of the oesophagus, the most common tumours are squamous cell carcinomas, like the tumours of the head and neck region described on pages 133-41. As we go down the oesophagus, however, more and more of the tumours are typical adenocarcinomas (see page 28), pathologically similar to those of the stomach. It is this group, particularly those situated at the lowest level – the gastro-oesophageal junction – that seem to have increased in incidence most strikingly over the past few years.

OESOPHAGEAL CANCER KEY POINTS
Incidence: Approximately 6,000 cases each year.
Age: 99% of cases occur over 40 years.
Risk factors: smoking, alcohol.

symptoms and diagnosis

- The most common symptom is difficulty in swallowing, often with a sense of the food 'sticking' or lodging at a particular site.
- Most patients have lost a considerable amount of weight by the time they see their GP but there may be little to detect on examination.

The key investigation is either a barium swallow test, in which the patient is X-rayed while swallowing a radio-opaque fluid containing barium, or direct inspection (endoscopy) using a semi-rigid fibre-optic telescope, which allows the oesophagus to be viewed directly. The malignant ulcer typical of oesophageal cancer can often be seen and biopsied quite easily but the barium swallow may give better evidence as to the length of the constriction if it proves impossible to pass the instrument beyond the narrowing. A simple chest X-ray may show whether there is glandular enlargement from lymph node spread in the centre of the chest, and CT scanning is also useful.

MOST COMMON SYMPTOMS OF OESOPHAGEAL CANCER
Dysphagia 85%
Heartburn 80%
Weight loss 60%
Anaemia 50%
Reflux 50%
Vomiting 25%

treatment

Oesophageal cancer is extremely difficult to deal with. Many patients are in fragile health, and the tumour has often spread quite far up and down the cylindrical oesophagus.

SURGERY

Surgical removal is possible only in a small minority of cases, and is a very major operation, since such a lengthy portion of the oesophagus is removed that a portion of small bowel or the stomach itself has to be mobilised upwards, for reconstruction. The long-term results of surgery are not very good, and radiotherapy is often preferred as a better method of treatment: it doesn't have the early mortality (around 10%) associated with even the best standards of surgical care.

RADIOTHERAPY AND CHEMOTHERAPY

Most patients with oesophageal cancer are unsuitable for radical radio-therapy, i.e. radiation given to high dose with the intention of cure. Either they are too unfit, or there might already be evidence of tumour spread to the liver or other sites; or the tumour volume required can simply be too large for the patient to withstand a radical dose. Nonetheless, as with surgery, there are certainly cases where even an unpromising carcinoma of the oesophagus has, against all expectation, been cured, though this is unusual.

Although radiotherapy is generally given by external beam treat-ment, the oesophagus lends itself particularly well to the concept of brachytherapy, with the patient treated by a radioactive wire or tube, which can be left in place, sitting snugly against the tumour, for the desired length of time before being removed. Increasingly, it is now recognised that chemotherapy, given alongside the radiation therapy (as simultaneous or 'synchronous' treatment) adds considerably to the chance of success, though there is still a very long way to go with this particularly nasty tumour. Cure rates do seem to be improving though.

LASER THERAPY

A most welcome advance in the management of oesophageal cancer during the past ten years has been the advent of laser therapy, which has truly transformed the lives of many patients, including those with inoperable disease. By burning through the tumour, it can rapidly pro-vide a new channel for the food and liquid to pass through, removing the obstruction and recanalising the organ so that decent nutrition can once again be achieved, while the patient is considered for additional treatment.

Laser therapy is a marvellous method to help the patient start to swallow and eat again, but sadly isn't a fundamental anti-cancer treat-ment. Unlike radiotherapy, it cannot penetrate outside the oesophagus and therefore has no place in the management of the more extensive portion of the tumour, within the wall of the oesophagus itself, or beyond, into the local nodal areas. It is, however, highly complement-ary with radiotherapy, and the two can be used together.

Laser therapy has provided the greatest advance in the symptomatic management of oesophageal cancer over the past 20 years, though overall cure rates remain poor, despite the much-improved palliation that can now be achieved quite regularly.

GASTRIC (STOMACH) CANCER

Cancers of the stomach have reduced sharply in incidence over the past 30 years, possibly due to improvements in our diet and reduction in smoking rates. Once again, a dietary causation is suggested by the dif-fering rates of prevalence of this tumour in different parts of the world.

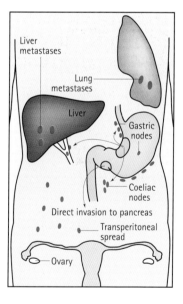

Common paths of spread in gastric (stomach) cancer.

causes

STOMACH CANCER KEY POINTS

Incidence:
Approximately 10,000 cases each year.

Age:
99% of cases occur over 40 years; 90% of gastric cancers occur over 55 years; the chance of a dyspeptic patient under the age of 55 having gastric cancer is one in a million.

Risk factors:
smoking, alcohol.

In Japan, for instance, it is so common that regular screening by fibre-optic direct vision techniques is widely performed. Environmental causes are suggested by the fact that within a generation or two, Japanese migrants to the United States show a reduction in incidence though still retaining a higher risk than the local indigenous population. The likelihood of developing gastric cancer is also related to socio-economic grouping (possibly through the smoking link), the disease being twice as common with increasing levels of deprivation. Although a nutritional or dietary cause of stomach cancer has long been considered likely, the nature of the offending substance(s) remains unclear.

● It is widely thought that green vegetables are protective, possibly by providing high levels of antioxidants, which prevent the process of carcinogenesis (cancer production or development).

● The same may also be true of vitamin C.

● A healthy diet, rich in fresh fruit and vegetables and low in dietary fats, offers the best means of avoiding this disease; non-smokers are also at much lower risk.

● The recognition of a link between a potentially pathological organism, Helicobacter pylori, and stomach malignancy has highlighted the importance of research spanning both the clinic and the lab; it looks as though Helicobacter pylori infection may be an extremely important contributor to– or even the cause of – stomach cancers, particularly the lymphomatous variety.

symptoms and diagnosis

Because of the rich lymphatic supply in and around the stomach, the tumour tends to spread early to local lymph nodes in the abdomen. Together with early evidence of blood-borne metastasis (most frequently to the liver), this often makes surgical treatment unsuitable for many patients. The most common symptoms include:

● Abdominal discomfort.

● Dyspepsia or indigestion (though a benign stomach or duodenal ulcer is far more common than any malignant process).

● Lethargy and loss of appetite.

● Patients often feel bloated, even after a small intake of food, and over-the-counter antacids don't generally help.

● Quite often, there is a substantial abdominal mass which can be felt by the GP or specialist, though this is generally less apparent to the patient himself.

Once again, the important investigations include a barium meal test and direct inspection using the fibre-optic gastroscope.

MOST COMMON SYMPTOMS OF STOMACH CANCER

Epigastric pain 90%
Weight loss 60%
Anaemia 50%
Loss of appetite 40%
Vomiting 25%

treatment

The treatment of gastric cancer should be surgical whenever possible. If the growth is limited to a particular part of the stomach, a 'partial gastrectomy' may be possible, but the larger the tumour, the less likely this is. A total gastrectomy, i.e. complete removal of the stomach, has much more serious consequences for the patient. As the stomach is so difficult to reconstruct, more extensive gastrectomy procedures with major lymph node dissection and removal, seem to give little if any additional benefit overall. On the other hand, patients who have inoperable cancer of the stomach gain little relief from local radiotherapy, which hasn't much to offer in this condition (though there are of course exceptions). This is partly because the stomach is surrounded by so many vital organs that the radiation dose is necessarily limited, and partly because of their relatively poor intrinsic responsiveness. Chemotherapy is more valuable, though there is no clear evidence that early (adjuvant) chemotherapy is helpful in cancers of the stomach, so its use remains limited to symptomatic palliation for inoperable or relapsed cases, where it can be useful.

LIVER CANCER

causes

Primary cancer of the liver is unusual in the Western world, but is much more common in parts of Africa. The cases that are seen in Europe arise most frequently in patients with chronic alcoholic damage to the liver (cirrhosis), or who have cirrhosis from another cause such as chronic viral hepatitis.

symptoms and diagnosis

- Clinically, most patients have either an obvious abdominal mass (generally right-sided) or jaundice, sometimes abdominal pain as well.
- Many have substantial distension from the malignant fluid (ascites) produced by the tumour.
- Far more common is the development of secondary hepatic (liver) deposits from a primary site elsewhere, most commonly a cancer of the large bowel (see page 110). The clinical features tend to be the same as for a primary liver tumour.

In both types, blood tests to assess liver function can give an idea of the likely outcome, though the general outlook is gloomy. In patients with secondary liver cancer, the simplest and least complicated means of diagnosis is ultrasound scanning, which is safe, reliable and easily repeated without any side-effects.

treatment

Patients with primary cancer of the liver are sometimes suitable for surgery, with removal of the diseased part. Liver transplantation is also gaining ground, though as with so many transplant programmes, there is a considerable shortage of organs for donation.

Even with secondary deposits within the liver, it is sometimes possible for the surgeon to remove these if circumstances are favourable, i.e. one or two deposits, in a restricted and accessible part of the organ.

On the whole, though, this applies only to a small minority, and treatment with chemotherapy (the details depending on the site of the primary tumour) is far more likely to be recommended.

Newer techniques include a direct attack on the secondary deposits by laser or radiofrequency ablation, using needles inserted through the skin, directly into the liver itself.

PANCREATIC CANCER

causes

Pancreatic cancer, a tumour with a high mortality rate, is unfortunately rising in incidence, though the reasons aren't clear. The time-scale of this rise has exactly paralleled the equivalent fall in gastric cancer incidence over the past 40 years.

● Pancreatic cancer is slightly more prevalent in men, occurring at a peak age of 55 to 60 years, and is twice as common in patients with diabetes.

● It also occurs more frequently in smokers and people who drink heavily.

MOST COMMON SYMPTOMS OF PANCREATIC CANCER
Jaundice 80%

symptoms and diagnosis

The majority of these tumours are, once again, adenocarcinomas (see page 28). Although many people associate the pancreas with insulin production (whose deficiency is the essential cause of diabetes), an equally important function of the pancreas is the manufacture of other digestive enzymes, which help break down food. These fluids are discharged into the bowel through the pancreatic duct, the pancreas itself lying in such close apposition to the liver and gall bladder that a tumour in the head of the pancreas (the most common site) almost always produces jaundice as well as abdominal pain.

treatment

Unfortunately, most of these tumours are already inoperable at the time of diagnosis, by virtue of widespread local extension to vital organ and lymph node groups. Surgery is, therefore, of limited benefit in pancreatic cancer, and, if carried out at all, has to be a very substantial procedure, performed by a specialist abdominal surgeon. Once again, the alternative, regrettably, is of minimal active treatment or the use of radiotherapy (with or without chemotherapy), which may be helpful symptomatically but won't be curative. Cancers of the pancreas are therefore among the most distressing of tumours, since so little can be done, yet they frequently arise in relatively fit patients below the age of 60 years. The outlook is poor, with radical surgical removal offering the only real hope of cure, and a five-year survival no greater than 15 per cent. On the other hand, palliative surgery by performing a by-pass between the up- and downstream parts of the bowel can be extremely helpful, even though there is no attempt to remove the tumour itself.

By-passing the tumour obstruction does at least improve the

PANCREATIC CANCER KEY POINTS
Incidence: Approximately 6,000 cases each year.
Age: 99% of cases occur over 40 years.
Risk factors: smoking, alcohol.

ALBERT'S STORY

Albert was 56 when his symptoms began, 58 when cancer of the pancreas was diagnosed and 59 when he died. He had noticed back pain for a month or two, but was a stoical sort of fellow and simply put up with it. His wife badgered him to see the doctor, but he wasn't keen. 'Indigestion,' he said.

However, after three more weeks of sleepless nights with Albert propped up in bed and clearly losing weight, she lost patience and got the GP round. Albert wasn't at all pleased and, out of spite, deliberately dropped cigarette ash over the bedclothes. The doctor was worried, but couldn't examine Albert properly, as he was too ill to move. The GP therefore arranged for a home visit by the local hospital specialist. He was also worried. 'Look at it this way, Albert,' he said, 'If it really is indigestion, it's pretty severe and hasn't responded to antacids and Tagamet; if it's just back pain, it would have got better by now; if it's something really serious, the sooner we know, the better.'

That really did scare Albert, but he was a stubborn man and only agreed to go into hospital after another week of relentless pleading by his wife. In hospital, the specialist's suspicions were strengthened; he hadn't been able to examine Albert properly at home, but it was easier in the hospital bed, and he was in little doubt that he could feel a firm abdominal mass. A CT scan and needle biopsy confirmed his suspicions – cancer of the pancreas. As with most cases, it was clearly inoperable, at least from the point of view of total tumour resection, by virtue of its close association with unresectable surrounding structures. 'Not good news, I'm afraid,' said the surgeon. 'Perhaps I'd be better off at home, then,' said Albert.

On the morning of his planned discharge three days later, when the pain was finally under control with regular long-acting morphine, they noticed for the first time a tinge of jaundice. By the time of Albert's first follow-up visit two weeks later, the jaundice was obvious to all. 'I'm afraid we'll have to get you back in to do a by-pass,' said the surgeon. 'If you want to do an operation, why didn't you do it first time around?' asked Albert. A further three weeks went by, the jaundice deepening almost every day, before he agreed to be re-admitted. By this time, the pain had become more severe, despite the long-acting morphine, and a team of Macmillan nurses had been called in by his GP. Perhaps it was too late.

As it turned out, the operation was rather more of a success than anyone had dared hope. Albert had become so itchy with the jaundice that it was more than just a cosmetic relief when it started to clear within days of the operation. The Macmillan team supervised the pain control with expert efficiency, and just over two weeks later, he was at home with his wife. He knew he was going to die, but it took longer than expected. They'd all wanted him to die at home, though eventually his wife had her doubts – she just wasn't sure whether she'd cope or not, even with the help available. 'I keep trying to imagine what it'll be like at the end, but I can't quite manage it.' 'You'll cope, don't worry, you'll cope,' said the Macmillan nurse.

Albert's wife was magnificent. She turned out to be more of a coper than she had dreamed possible. Most of the time, the Macmillan team stayed in the background, but it was good to know that they were always contactable. She and Albert hadn't been great talkers, but suddenly they found themselves more in tune than before. He wasn't a religious man, he said, but he wanted to get a few things off his chest. 'He actually apologised to me for all that f'ing and blinding when he used to go out drinking,' she said, after he had died. 'I was angry with him for bringing that up when the truth was far worse – women, gambling, the lot. But I suppose I loved him all the same – and I was pleased I could look after him until the end.'

symptoms for a while, giving the patient and family a breathing space, at least, to help come to terms with the disease. In some patients, it may be possible to deal with the obstruction without a major operation, by means of an internal 'stenting' procedure, whereby a semi-rigid tube (the stent) is placed into the obstructed duct using a cunning endoscopic approach, passing the instrument all the way down through the oesophagus, stomach, duodenum (the first part of the small bowel) and directly into the blocked area. This ingenious technique is often effective for several months, and at least avoids the hazards of radical surgical procedures. Pain control can be a real problem with these tumours, but radiotherapy can be helpful and proper attention to use of analgesics (pain killers) or nerve blocks can make all the difference.

BOWEL CANCER

Cancer of the small bowel is fortunately very rare. Less than one in 20 of all gastro-intestinal tumours occur at this site, which seems rather odd, since the small bowel is so lengthy. By contrast, tumours of the large bowel are among the most common in the Western world and represent the second largest cause of cancer death. The fact that the disease is unusual in large parts of Africa, Asia and South America suggests a possible dietary cause, and there seems little doubt that cancer of the large bowel is far more common in populations with a high intake of meat products and a relatively low level of dietary fibre. Reducing the intake of meat and animal fat and increasing dietary fibre (particularly with plenty of green vegetables) are an important means of reducing the incidence of these cancers. The commonest sites for these cancers are in the colon and, still lower down, the rectum – the lowest part of the bowel, which leads directly to the anus.

BOWEL CANCER KEY POINTS

Incidence:
Approximately 30,000 cases
each year.

Age:
99% of cases occur over 40 years.
85% of cases occur over 60 years.

causes

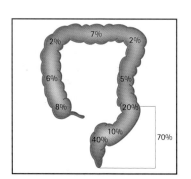

Distribution of colorectal cancer, by
large bowel site.

● Although initially laughed out of court, the surgeon and epidemiologist Sir Denis Burkitt, branded as over-obsessional with the dietary and bowel habits of rural Africans, showed quite clearly that the disease was rare in this population because of the rapid rate of digested food passing through their bowel. This gives far less opportunity for a potential carcinogen to remain in contact with a particular part of the bowel surface for a significant length of time.
● Hereditary conditions are also known to predispose to bowel cancer, including the non-cancerous but potentially pre-malignant condition of ulcerative colitis, a relapsing large bowel disorder, in which bowel involvement can be extensive.
● Young patients with this disorder are at particular risk of developing bowel cancer, so much so that, in the past, some physicians recommended total removal of the bowel (total colectomy) to avoid the risk.
● Nowadays, careful regular screening and follow-up using fibre-optic

colonoscopy have largely replaced this extreme recommendation. In this procedure, a flexible telescope can be introduced at the anus and passed carefully up through the whole of the large bowel, in order to give a direct view and, where necessary, allow a biopsy of any suspicious site.

● In familial polyposis, a separate condition characterised by multiple benign polyps of the bowel, there is also a predisposition to malignant change, particularly in the lower half of the colon, and preventive or 'prophylactic' surgery is sometimes recommended in this group.

● As for prevention, a number of studies have suggested that regular use of non-steroidal anti-inflammatory drugs such as aspirin or ibuprofen (Brufen, Nurofen) may be beneficial, though the side-effect of gastro-intestinal bleeding remains a serious drawback.

● Benign (non-familial) polyps of the large bowel are extremely common, and discussion has raged for many years as to whether or not they are genuinely pre-malignant. Bowel polyps are discovered increasingly with advancing age, and only a small percentage become malignant, though evidence of a previously benign-looking polyp is sometimes found close by the malignant tumour in the surgical specimen, raising the question of whether or not an originally benign polyp might have become more aggressive. Large polyps carry a greater risk than smaller ones and should certainly be removed.

> **FACTORS AFFECTING THE RISK OF BOWEL CANCER**
>
> *Increased risk*
> ● Probable: high consumption of red and processed meat.
>
> ● Possible: high fat consumption, obesity, high alcohol consumption.
>
> *Decreased risk*
> ● Probable: high fibre consumption, high vegetable consumption, high level of physical activity.
>
> ● Possible: high fruit consumption, nonsteroidal anti-inflammatory drugs including aspirin.

symptoms and diagnosis

● Most patients with cancer of the bowel have a fairly obvious change in bowel habit, i.e. constipation and/or diarrhoea.

● The precise position of the tumour within the large bowel often dictates the nature of other symptoms such as pain, rectal bleeding or weight loss.

● Tumours of the right side (ascending colon) tend to cause more in the way of abdominal pain than left-sided (descending colon) or rectal tumours, whereas, perhaps not surprisingly, cancers of the rectum present far more commonly with bleeding.

● Complete obstruction, with inability to open the bowels at all (often with persistent vomiting and discomfort), occurs in about 10% of cases.

● Rectal bleeding may be obvious, with fresh, bright-red blood mixed into the stool, but tumours from higher up the bowel are more likely to cause blackened stools, because the blood has become chemically altered by the time it appears in the expelled stools.

● The pain of colonic cancer is typically colicky, coming and going, intermittent, sometimes rising to a severe cramp-like crescendo.

These symptoms require urgent attention and evaluation. A rectal examination by the family doctor or specialist will often be sufficient to suggest the diagnosis though, obviously, tumours higher in the bowel are well beyond the reach of the examining finger. Rapid referral to a hospital specialist is extremely important, since early detection and treatment are the key to success.

> **MOST COMMON SYMPTOMS OF BOWEL CANCER**
>
> Intermittent or persistent rectal bleeding.
>
> Change in bowel habit – most commonly increased frequency and/or looser stools persistent for at least six weeks.

The investigations will include a sigmoidoscopy: the insertion of a rigid tube, with proper illumination and biopsy attachments, into the rectum and lowest part of the colon. This gives rapid diagnosis in a large proportion of colorectal tumours, since well over half are situated in the rectum or sigmoid – again, suggesting that food carcinogens are the cause of these tumours, since this part of the bowel is the final depot for digested food particles before defecation.

Other important investigations include the barium enema (in which a tube is inserted into the anus and radio-opaque barium dye passed as a liquid up into the bowel) but increasingly patients with suspicious symptoms are investigated with colonoscopy and CT scanning. In this technique, both air and contrast material are used to give even clearer images of the tumour and its likely pattern of spread.

treatment

These tumours are mostly typical adenocarcinomas (see page 28), and the two important pathological features are the degree of invasion from the inside of the bowel wall (the mucosa or lining) through the muscular coating of the bowel to the outer surface (the serosa), and whether or not there is lymph node involvement in the resected bowel specimen. This type of surgical staging has stood the test of time and is known to be the most important indicator of outcome.

SURGERY

Most patients with early-stage bowel cancers, confined to the lining, are cured by surgery, though the margins of clearance have to be sufficiently generous. So cancers of the ascending colon are often dealt with by removing the whole of the right-hand portion of the large bowel (a right hemicolectomy), and tumours of the descending and upper sigmoid colon by a left hemicolectomy (the same, but on the left side). Fortunately, there is sufficient redundancy in the human intestine that we can do perfectly well with only half the large bowel; the outcome is generally excellent, with careful joining (anastomosis) of the cut ends of the bowel, and no permanent need for a colostomy.

Cancers of the lower bowel, however, including many rectal carcinomas, will generally require either a temporary or permanent colostomy, in which the upper cut end of the bowel is brought out on to the abdominal wall, with a stoma and a collecting bag for the stools, rather than attempting a dangerous anastomosis at the lowest rectal or anal level, for fear that the operation will be insufficiently generous to clear the cancer completely.

RADIOTHERAPY AND CHEMOTHERAPY

A cancer that has penetrated a significant portion of the bowel musculature, or broken through to the outside or to local lymph nodes, is much more difficult to control by surgery alone. Fortunately, it became

LIVING WITH A COLOSTOMY

Obviously, it is always disappointing for patients to hear that they may need a colostomy, but for many, it will be the price of a permanent cure. Although many are naturally worried about the appearance of a colostomy and the possibility of constant embarrassment, social isolation, spillage and smell, most are also worried that they will find it impossible to manage the colostomy themselves without skilled help. They need encouragement, support and reassurance that the presence of the colostomy does not imply that part of the cancer has been left behind, or that it will prove impossible to return to a normal active life.

Many patients faced with the possibility of a permanent colostomy find it helpful to meet others who have undergone this procedure and have learned to cope with it, before facing surgery themselves. They, in turn, are then sometimes called on to counsel other patients, and may gain considerable self-esteem from making this contribution to the welfare of others. Although some patients take many months to come to terms with a colostomy, the majority find it far less difficult and degrading than they might have expected. Many hospitals have stoma therapy clinical nurse specialists, able to educate, counsel and support patients with colostomies. Self-help groups (see useful addresses on page 216) are also extremely active in this field. A colostomy may need to be permanent or only temporary, depending on the precise nature and site of the tumour.

increasingly clear through the 1990s that both chemotherapy and radiotherapy had a part to play. Early (adjuvant) use of chemotherapy, i.e. immediately after surgery, without waiting for a recurrence, can improve the outcome in these more advanced tumours, even though the additional benefit may be rather limited at present, since currently available anti-cancer agents are not yet powerful enough in bowel cancer.

Post-operative radiotherapy for locally advanced large bowel cancers is limited to rectal tumours, but can be extremely valuable in preventing local recurrence. It is this danger, together with the risk of more widespread involvement, that represents the greatest threat to the health of a patient who has successfully undergone surgery for cancer of the bowel.

As for metastatic involvement to the liver, it is a curious fact that this unwelcome eventuality, though always regrettable, does not always imply rapid progression and early death. For some reason, a proportion of patients with liver deposits from rectal or colonic carcinomas can live for many months or even years with the appropriate treatment – generally chemotherapy, but, just occasionally, surgical removal of the secondary deposits or laser therapy (still an experimental technique) if limited to a particular part of the liver.

Bowel cancers at the lowest level of all, the anus, have increased in frequency during recent years, though they still only account for a tiny proportion of large bowel cancers. Until a few years ago, anal cancer was slightly more common in women, but it appears to be an HIV-related malignancy and certainly became more common in homosexual men during the 1980s. It is generally treated by radiotherapy and synchro-

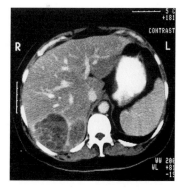

CT scan showing a large hepatic metastasis (i.e. a secondary deposit in the liver) seen as a dark grey area at bottom left. The bowel cancer had been removed two years before.

nous chemotherapy in order to preserve the anal sphincter and, as far as possible, normal bowel function without colostomy. Surgical resection, which always requires colostomy, will be required for patients who fail this initial treatment. However, only a few years ago, all patients with anal cancer were recommended for this type of surgery, so this welcome change towards non-surgical treatment represents a real step in the right direction. There is a far smaller probability of colostomy being required, as a result of failure of control at the primary site, with the combination therapy using chemo- and radiotherapy together.

MILDRED'S STORY

Mildred had been constipated for as long as she could remember, but couldn't ever recall it being quite this bad. Divorced ten years previously, and now aged 71, she had struggled to get her life back together after a rather bitter marriage lasting almost 30 years and producing two children that she did not like; she was, in truth, shut off from her family and the rest of the world around her.

She was embarrassed to go to her GP, but felt she had to. The GP thought she could feel something odd with the tip of her examining finger, so she sent Mildred off to the local specialist, who saw her after a six-week gap. By this time, the rectal carcinoma was a little bigger, and the surgeon had no difficulty confirming its presence with a sigmoidoscopy and barium enema. She was hopeful that it could be resected without the need for a permanent colostomy.

In the event, Mildred was relatively lucky and no permanent colostomy was needed, but unfortunately that wasn't the end of the matter. Although the surgeon had found no evidence of tumour dissemination within the abdomen, the pathologist later confirmed that there was, indeed, significant evidence of spread through the bowel wall and explained as much to her surgical colleague at their monthly conference, with the slides projected on to a screen. The surgeon sought the opinion of the radiotherapist, since surgery alone was clearly not very likely to cure the patient.

The radiotherapist explained the wide variety of opinion, but said that, in her own view, the sensible course of action would be to have both radiotherapy and chemotherapy, 'to be on the safe side.' Mildred did extremely well with this treatment, although the temporary painful skin reaction during radiotherapy, particularly between her buttocks, was more uncomfortable than she had bargained for. Most of the staff had warned her that the chemotherapy was likely to be worse, but, with her, it was the other way round.

Eighteen months later, they told her that one of the blood tests they had been using to monitor her progress had shown a slight rise in one of the marker levels (it was the CEA test, see opposite) and a further scan would have to be done. Sadly, this showed evidence of two small secondary cancer deposits within the liver, and these would have to be dealt with by laser, surgery or chemotherapy. Mildred was reasonably happy to leave the decision to the experts, and, in the end, a combination of all three techniques was felt to offer the best chance of success.

Twelve months on, she has now completed the whole of the planned treatment, all of which went well. In the end, she lost about a third of her liver, leaving her quite sufficient to get by on, and she's now been off treatment for six months with no evidence of a further rise in the CEA. In the meantime, Mildred seems to have blossomed. Having decided that one of her two children isn't quite as unappealing as she had thought, having done the decent thing and produced two grandchildren for her to inspect, she took herself off to visit them in Australia. She'd never flown before.

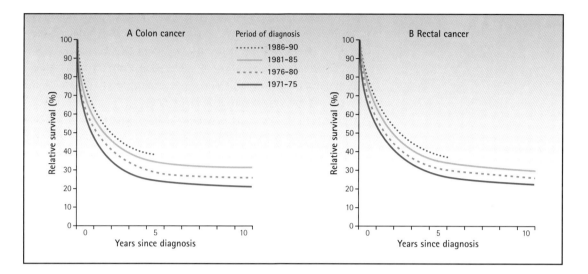

More than 80% of patients with early carcinomas confined to the mucosa, survive for at least five years, and the majority of these patients prove, in the long run, to have been cured by surgery. Where there has been involvement of the muscle of the bowel wall, the figure falls to about 50%. Even lymph node involvement can be associated with lengthy survival and probable cure if the nodes have all been resected and the surgery supplemented by radio- and/or chemotherapy. There is no doubt that surgery remains the absolute cornerstone of treatment – non-surgical approaches, though extremely valuable in selected cases, will not be replacing surgery in the foreseeable future.

Large bowel tumours do sometimes produce a tumour marker known as CEA (carcino-embryonic antigen) and detectable by a blood test which, although not specific to bowel cancer, can be a valuable means of following progress. Such markers can help cancer specialists to identify a probable recurrence before the patient has developed symptoms, while it is still surgically operable. It's not yet clear whether the routine use of CEA monitoring will improve overall survival results; this is another area of current study by a randomised controlled trial.

Relative survival (%) for colon and rectal cancer in England and Wales, in adults diagnosed 1971-1990. The graphs show the continuous improvement in survival over this 20-year period.

GENITO-URINARY CANCERS

Cancers of the kidney, bladder, prostate and penis (see the following pages) are an extremely important group, accounting for over a quarter of all cancers in men. Within these so-called genito-urinary cancers, kidney (renal) tumours are by far the least common. As far as causation is concerned, there are only a few rather sketchy clues.

● For tumours of the kidney, there is at least one congenital syndrome (a disease known as von Hippel-Lindau syndrome, characterised by

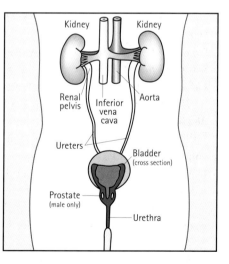

Diagram of the urinary tract showing the anatomy of the main structures (excluding the penis).

spongy blood vessel overgrowths in parts of the brain), which happens to be quite common. In the outflow part of the kidney, the collecting system that drains off the urine, tumours occur that are different from the most common variety of cancer of the kidney, the adenocarcinoma.
● Both renal and bladder tumours are more prevalent in smokers or ex-smokers and are much more common in men (about three to one for cancer of the kidney and six to one for bladder cancer).

symptoms and diagnosis

Symptoms are generally related to the formation and passage of urine.
● The most common symptom is bleeding into the urine.
● Pain can be a feature, though even large kidney tumours can be surprisingly painless.

RICHARD'S STORY

Richard had just turned 50 when he developed low back pain and weakness of the legs. He saw his GP, who said it was a disc and laid him off work for a fortnight. However, as a self-employed travelling sales-man, it was costing him money and, in any event, he wasn't much better after a week, so he simply got on with his life and took Nurofen for the pain. A month later, Richard collapsed in the street when his legs buckled under him, and a passing cab driver brought him into his local casualty department where an X-ray confirmed almost total destruction of the lowest two lumbar vertebrae. There was no clue as to what might be the cause, and general examination was normal apart from his grossly weakened legs, so a biopsy was performed by one of the orthopaedic surgeons.

A week later, the pathologists reported undoubted malignancy, but they were quite certain that the lumbar vertebrae were a secondary rather than the primary site, since the microscopic appearances didn't correspond to any of the known primary cancers of the bone. Could this be a cancer of the kidney, they wondered? Sure enough, the abdominal ultrasound confirmed a substantial primary cancer of the right kidney, measuring almost 10 centimetres across, which, despite its size, had not previously declared itself. An isotope bone scan had already been done, and no other secondary deposits were seen.

It was clear that Richard ought to have a course of palliative radiotherapy to the lower spine, and, for-tunately, his pain improved a good deal, although he still required the long-acting morphine tablets prescribed after the diagnosis had first been made. Radiotherapy reduced his morphine requirement by about two-thirds. He was also referred to a urologist, in case there was any advantage in removing the kidney, but he thought not, so radiotherapy is the only form of active treatment Richard has had.

Eighteen months have now gone by, and he's doing pretty well. The real problem, though, is that, despite his happy-go-lucky character, his wife simply can't cope with the uncertainty of it all. Although not burdened with guilt about her own good health and his infirmity (as many are), she's constantly close to the edge with a degree of anxiety that rarely leaves and counselling hasn't helped. For Richard, strug-gling on with an incurable disease currently under control, her inability to support him (or even cope with her own distress) is the most exhausting aspect of the illness. He feels cheated that he, the patient, is expected to be the strong one. He finds it easier to cope with the uncertainty and lack of treatment than she does, and his best hope is that further counselling will help her to develop the skill she needs to learn how to stop driving him crazy with her constant, well-meant attentions and cross-questioning.

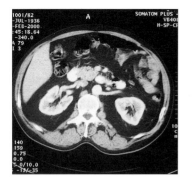
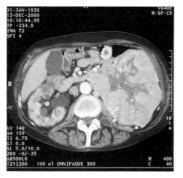

Cancer of the kidney (renal carcinoma). The left image shows normal anatomy. In the right image, the normal left kidney is totally replaced by a massive tumour. The patient had surprisingly few symptoms and had survived for more than three years.

● With the less commonly encountered cancers of the kidney, there are symptoms of secondary spread, since they metastasise to bone.

treatment

Cancers of the kidney should be dealt with by surgery if at all possible. We only need one kidney, so it is perfectly feasible and technically correct to remove the whole of the kidney (nephrectomy) if a renal cancer is discovered. The ureter is often removed as well (and is certainly not much use anyway, without the kidney). Although this may cure the cancer, some renal tumours are locally very advanced and cure cannot be guaranteed, even with removal of the whole kidney.

These tumours do have a reputation for late dissemination, notably to bone and lung, so careful follow-up is important. In patients with disease beyond the initial site, nephrectomy may still be sensible if the primary tumour is causing real discomfort or other symptoms. In this respect, renal cancer is unusual – surgery in the face of widespread disease wouldn't make much sense. There are even cases on record in which removal of the primary tumour has resulted in shrinkage of secondary deposits, though it isn't known why this occasionally occurs. An alternative is to 'embolise' the tumour, a technique devised with the specific intent of aiming to shrink the tumour with an injection of occlusive material, directly into the renal artery, which gives the kidney its blood supply.

MOST COMMON SYMPTOMS OF KIDNEY CANCER
Blood in urine Loin pain Renal masses Anaemia Weight loss Fever

BLADDER CANCER

causes

For bladder cancers, rather more is known about causation than for cancer of the kidney. In the UK, it is the sixth most common cause of cancer death in men.

● By the end of the nineteenth century, it was recognised that workers in the aniline dye industry had a high incidence of this type of cancer, and it later became clear that this was due to a carcinogen, a cancer-promoting substance, produced during the dye-production process.

● Other occupational groups have also been recognised as being at risk, notably those in the rubber and cable industries.

● Bladder cancer is also reportedly more common in urban than rural areas, and one other predisposing feature, of great significance in the Middle East, is the chronic bladder inflammation caused by schistosomiasis, an infection resulting from a burrowing fluke which chronically infests the bladder wall, entering the body by a water-borne route, chiefly from polluted rivers or streams.

symptoms and diagnosis

● In bladder cancer, the most common symptom is bleeding into the urine. This is usually painless, though many patients have symptoms such as urgency of micturition (a very strong desire to pass urine), nocturia (passing urine at night) and frequency of micturition or reduction of the urinary stream.

Although patients with frequency of micturition and discomfort may simply be suffering from cystitis, persistent symptoms will require investigation. If examination reveals an obvious mass in the abdomen or side of the body (loin), the quickest confirmatory test is usually an ultrasound scan followed by CT or MRI imaging.

In patients with haematuria, the urologist will arrange for cystoscopy, a simple and informative investigation in which a narrow tube (cystoscope) is passed under anaesthetic directly through the penis into the bladder, giving very good direct vision of the whole of the bladder's interior surface. This will often reveal one or more areas of tumour; in some cases, a substantial portion of the bladder lining (mucosa) is involved. Cystoscopic biopsy will also reveal the extent to which the tumour has penetrated from the bladder lining into the muscular wall. This is a most important pathological feature that has considerable prognostic weight.

MOST COMMON SYMPTOMS OF BLADDER CANCER

Blood in urine
Strong and frequent desire to urinate
Mass in the abdomen

treatment

HEAT APPLICATION AND CHEMOTHERAPY

For relatively superficial tumours within the bladder, the use of local heat application ('diathermy') to burn the tumours away is often very effective, but may have to be repeated on a number of occasions.

If the tumours are larger or more extensive, chemotherapy can be given directly into the bladder, again on repeated occasions. In any event, virtually all patients with bladder cancer require repeat cystoscopy at regular intervals, to monitor progress – generally under a short anaesthetic as a day case.

RADIOTHERAPY AND/OR SURGERY

For more deeply situated bladder tumours the risk of dissemination to other parts of the body (local lymph nodes, lung, liver and bone) is considerably greater, and cystodiathermy and intravesical chemotherapy (i.e. direct instillation into the bladder) are insufficient. Either radiotherapy or removal of the bladder will be necessary. Both are effective, but, treatment by radical radiotherapy has become more widely employed as few patients would willingly lose the bladder, with the inevitable consequence of requiring a new route for urine flow. If required, this is generally achieved by means of an ileal conduit, formed from a short portion of bowel, with the ureters implanted directly into it and brought out on to the abdominal wall with a permanent stoma and collecting bag.

Fortunately, radical radiotherapy for deeply penetrating bladder tumours is frequently effective, although a cure can never be guaranteed. It has the enormous advantage of preservation of the bladder, and if local recurrence does occur, it is generally possible to consider total cystectomy at a later stage. Few bladder tumours are treatable by partial removal of the bladder because the disease is often quite widespread over the bladder surface. The treatment of deeply invading bladder cancer lies between radical radiotherapy and radical surgery. If patients are to be considered for either, pelvic scanning is essential to determine the limits of the tumour, since, not uncommonly, evidence of extra-vesical spread (i.e. outside the bladder) will be discovered.

Although most patients are happier with the prospect of facing radical radiotherapy rather than surgery, the treatment course can be quite tough. It lasts between three and six weeks, depending on local practice, and may produce uncomfortable urinary symptoms as a result of the effect of the X-ray beam directly on the bladder lining. Urinary frequency and nocturia can persist long after the course of treatment. Repeat cystoscopy will be required to ascertain whether or not the treatment has been successful. In some patients, the radiotherapy appears to shrink the bladder permanently, with the probability of more frequent micturition (including at night-time) as a long-term consequence of cure.

OTHER TREATMENTS

For more superficial tumours of the bladder lining, new treatments are coming in all the time. Apart from cystodiathermy, treatment by extreme freezing (cryosurgery) and laser are also possible, and there is quite a range of suitable intra-vesical chemotherapy agents. Instillation of BCG (the agent often used to immunise against tuberculosis during childhood) directly into the bladder is also effective in slowing down the rate of progression.

It is important to stress that treatment of urological malignancies can be consistent with a remarkably normal quality of life. The many competing treatments now available – including surgery, radiotherapy and chemotherapy – mean that many patients have to find their way through quite a complex treatment maze. Although many are in late middle age or beyond, age per se should never be a reason to compromise treatment intensity, particularly where cure is a realistic possibility.

prognosis

> **BLADDER CANCER KEY POINTS**
>
> - 12,000 cases each year in England and Wales.
>
> - Most often occurs in the 65 to 80 years age group.
>
> - Men more likely to be affected than women by 3 to 1.

PROSTATE CANCER

Very little is known about the causation of cancer of the prostate, though it is among the most common of all male cancers (second after lung), increasing in incidence directly with advancing age. It is even thought possible that all men who live long enough will develop it, though not necessarily as a clinical problem during life.

- In the United States, it is the third most common cause of cancer death in males, exceeded only by lung and large bowel cancers.
- US figures also show a much higher mortality rate in blacks than whites, and it is one of several malignancies that appear to have become more common in the second half of the twentieth century.
- It is clearly hormone dependent, requiring testosterone (the male hormone produced in the testicles) for its continued growth, never occurring in men who have been castrated.
- In recent years, the importance of family clustering has begun to be recognised in prostate cancer, though most cases appear to have no very obvious genetic background.

PROSTATE CANCER KEY POINTS

- 16,000 cases each year in England and Wales.
- 99% of cases occur in men aged over 50 years.
- About 25% of cases present in men aged less than 70 years, when life expectancy is more than 10 years.

With cancer of the prostate, the discovery of the malignant tumour is usually an incidental finding at surgery for what was thought to be a benign prostatic enlargement – or, more accurately, after surgery, when the pathology report is available. Many elderly men require such surgery because enlargement of the prostate (far more commonly a benign than a malignant disorder) has caused obstruction of the urethra, producing difficulties with micturition as described above.

- It is often possible, though, to detect a prostate cancer simply by rectal examination, since the prostate gland, which can be felt via the rectum quite easily, often feels hard or craggy if malignant.
- Increasingly, annual examination is performed as a general screening measure, often including a rectal exam and blood test for PSA (prostate-specific antigen), a useful tumour marker discussed in more detail opposite. A rise in PSA in the non-symptomatic patient is becoming one of the more common means of diagnosis.
- A significant proportion of patients with prostatic cancer do, however, have symptoms of secondary spread, since this is relatively common, chiefly affecting the bones of the pelvis, hips and lower vertebral area. This also applies to the far less commonly encountered cancers of the kidney, since these also metastasise to bone.

For cancer of the prostate, generally an adenocarcinoma (see page 28), tumour staging is again important, since this dictates treatment as well as determining outcome. Ultrasound techniques are often used, with direct scanning of the prostate by means of the trans-rectal route, allowing the scanner tip to be placed in almost direct proximity to the prostate itself. In patients who seem likely to have a prostatic carcinoma detected before a trans-urethral resection procedure (TUR), a

---

MOST COMMON SYMPTOMS IN PROSTATE CANCER

Increased and persistent need to urinate

possibility often raised by discovery of an elevated PSA level, trans-rectal prostatic biopsy can be accomplished with minimal anaesthesia. As with bladder cancer, CT and MRI scanning will give important information as to the local extent of disease.

treatment

As far as management of prostate cancer is concerned, there are few areas in cancer where such diversity of opinion exists, even among experts. There isn't even complete agreement as to how treatment of early prostatic cancer should be undertaken – whether by surgery or radiotherapy – though most would nowadays agree that some attempt at curative therapy should be made.

HORMONE TREATMENTS

One alternative, hotly debated among specialists, is the use of hormone treatments, since it has been known for over 50 years that most prostatic cancers are hormonally dependent. Both oestrogen therapy (female hormones) and removal of both testicles (orchidectomy) have been known for decades to be useful for palliation, often benefiting patients who have widespread, painful bone disease from secondary prostate cancer. Since many patients, including all those with a positive bone scan at diagnosis, are unsuitable for radical surgery or radiotherapy, the use of these (and newer) hormone techniques has become increasingly accepted both for early and advanced cases.

For patients with more advanced disease, where there is no prospect of cure, hormone treatments offer the best chance of long-term palliation and symptom control, often working effectively for many months or years, with progress monitored by regular checks of PSA. There are many agents available, of which the most common are cyproterone (given in tablet form) and the most recently introduced goserelin, given as a monthly injection.

These work by reducing testosterone levels via an effect on the pituitary gland at the base of the brain – and they have replaced the old-fashioned approach with oestrogen, which could cause undesirable feminisation, including breast enlargement.

RADIOTHERAPY

In patients with localised disease, the choice lies between radical surgery (prostatectomy) and radical irradiation. Each has its advocates and surgery is performed very widely in the USA, perhaps less frequently in Britain. Because of the risks of incontinence and post-operative impotence through surgical nerve damage, radical radiation therapy is often preferred as the treatment of choice, though as with radical irradiation for bladder cancer, symptoms during and after prostatic radiation can be quite troublesome. This form of treatment is extremely effective for early, well-localised tumours, with many patients retaining normal

FACTORS AFFECTING THE RISK OF DEVELOPING PROSTATIC CANCER

Demographic
• Increasing age.
• Place of residence.

Genetic
• Family history of prostate cancer.
• Family history of breast cancer.
• Race – black.

Dietary
• High fat consumption.
• Low green vegetable consumption.

Occupational
• Cadmium exposure.
• Radiation exposure.
• Farming.

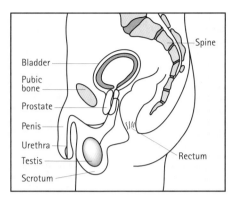

Diagram of the urinary tract showing the position of the prostate.

bladder functioning and sexual potency afterwards, unless adjuvant hormone therapy has also been recommended, in an attempt to reduce the male hormone (testosterone) levels to zero. Treatment with radioactive seed implants – directly into the prostate – is becoming popular though most oncological departments still prefer to practise conversional external beam irradiation.

SURGERY

In some cases where the disease is more advanced, treatment by orchidectomy is the only means of gaining control of the tumour. It is not, of course, a step that would ever be undertaken lightly but it is often accepted by these predominantly elderly patients extremely well.

prognosis Results of treatment for prostate cancer are unusually difficult to assess, because of its uncertain and often slow natural history together with the high death rate in any group of elderly men. About 50% of patients are alive after ten years, with better results where the disease was apparently limited to the prostate gland without evidence of local extension. Few patients with bone deposits survive in the long term, however, despite high initial response rates to hormone therapy, and chemotherapy has remained disappointing as a potential additional method of treatment, though it is certainly used, with benefit, in usually selected cases.

PENILE CANCER

Cancers of the penis are very uncommon. They tend to develop near the tip rather than the shaft, sometimes with a very slow period of evolution, over many years. In appearance, they may resemble an ulcer – though non-malignant ulcers are far more common. They tend to spread to the nodes in the groin (the inguinal area) and are treated either by radiotherapy or surgery, sometimes both. Usually they are fairly well localised, and radiotherapy can produce an excellent result with full healing and no further problems.

Surgery will be necessary, however, if the patient suffers a local recurrence; fortunately, it is often possible to perform local surgery without having to amputate the whole organ – and half a penis can work surprisingly well. However, involvement of the inguinal and other nodal areas makes complete cure much more difficult. Cancer of the penis often seems to run a slow, rather indolent course, with some patients appearing cured by the initial radiotherapy, but developing a local recurrence or inguinal lymph node disease several years after initial treatment.

TESTICULAR CANCER

Over the past century there has been a tenfold increase in the incidence of testicular cancer in industrialised nations, though no one quite knows why except for one or two important predisposing factors.

● The most important is the presence of an undescended testicle, a congenital abnormality which some boys are born with. The longer it is left in its incorrect position – generally in the abdomen or in the inguinal (groin) region, the greater is the risk of malignant change.

● Inflammation of the testes during a mumps episode (so-called mumps orchitis) may also predispose to testicular malignancy.

Before birth, the testicles are situated within the abdomen and pass through the inguinal canal in the groin to their final position. It may well be that the additional warmth of the abdominal environment is the stimulating factor in provoking malignant change, since the normal testicle is held at a much lower temperature, effectively outside the body, within the scrotum. Interestingly, in boys who have a single undescended testicle, it is not only this one, but the other, too, which is at increased risk of cancer in later life, so it really is of the utmost importance to perform a surgical correction of an undescended testis. There is a second reason, too: poorly descended testicles rarely produce sperm, so infertility is another likely consequence. Trauma to the testes is often implicated as a causative factor for cancer, but this is generally believed (by the medical profession, at any rate) to be false.

● The initial symptom is usually a painless testicular enlargement, though pain, sometimes of a dragging or throbbing type, is occasionally a feature.

● Some patients have back pain as well, sometimes from lymph node involvement in the pelvic or lower abdominal glands.

● When blood-borne spread takes place, it is generally to the lungs, though several other sites can be involved as well. In the celebrated recent case of the American cyclist Lance Armstrong, three-times winner of the Tour de France, the disease had even spread to the brain. He won his remarkable victories some years after successful treatment of testicular cancer by chemotherapy, and fathered children after chemotherapy as well: the sky's the limit! (We show him on page 38.)

Most testicular tumours are termed either seminoma or teratoma (though much more complicated terms are also used) depending on the particular type of malignancy, but the important fact is that they are tumours of the reproductive cells themselves – referred to generally as 'germ cell tumours'. Non-germ cell tumours, from the supporting structures of the testes, are much less common. This sets the testicular tumours apart, pathologically, from the other more common types of solid cancer, and their behaviour is very different too. Although they spread by the classical pathways of blood-borne, lymphatic and direct

causes

symptoms and diagnosis

TESTICULAR CANCER KEY POINTS
Incidence: 1,400 cases each year in England and Wales.
Age: Indeterminate swellings of the testicle have a low probability of being due to cancer, especially in men over 55 years and should be considered for ultrasound before urological referral.

MOST COMMON SYMPTOMS OF TESTICULAR CANCER
Solid scrotal swellings

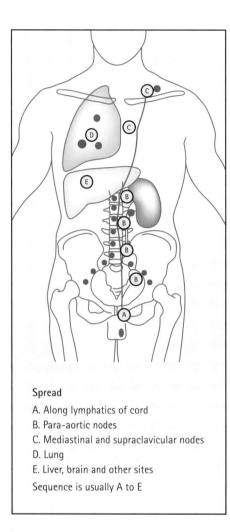

Spread

A. Along lymphatics of cord
B. Para-aortic nodes
C. Mediastinal and supraclavicular nodes
D. Lung
E. Liver, brain and other sites

Sequence is usually A to E

Typical pathways of dissemination in testicular cancer.

local extension, their response to radiotherapy and chemotherapy is markedly different from most solid tumours, and they are a highly curable group even if widely spread at the time of diagnosis.

Staging and surgical removal of the primary site are the important first steps and may be sufficient for localised cases. With chest X-ray, and thoracic plus abdominal scanning to supplement thorough clinical examination and marker studies (see below), most patients can be shown either to have localised disease or evidence of disease beyond the primary site, with various stages assigned to increasing degrees of involvement.

TUMOUR MARKERS

Testicular cancers also differ from most other tumours in another very important respect – the production and secretion into the bloodstream of tumour marker substances, which are directly produced by the tumour. The higher the marker level, the greater the amount of viable malignant tissue present. The two main marker substances are AFP (alpha fetoprotein) and HCG (human chorionic gonadotrophin). These are made by specific and different cells within the malignant tissue, some tumours producing one but not the other, though many producing both.

Measurement of these markers in the blood allows reliable pre-operative diagnosis even without biopsy, and is of immense value in follow-up. Successful treatment should lead to complete abolition, to virtually zero levels, of both of them. If after a period of normality one or other starts to rise, relapse is almost certain, even though the patient may feel completely well without any other supporting evidence of recurrent disease at that early stage. All this would be of academic interest only if there was no useful treatment for patients who are not cured by initial surgery. But fortunately this is not the case, since testicular germ cell tumours are among the most chemo-sensitive of all adult tumours, and in addition, the seminomas, which tend to affect a slightly older age group, are extremely responsive to radiotherapy as well.

treatment   Although uncommon, testicular tumours are the most important cause of cancer in men between the ages of 15 and 30 years. The overwhelming majority of patients are completely cured either by surgery alone (most stage 1 cases) or by surgery with post-operative chemotherapy. Removal of the whole testicle (orchidectomy) is recommended, and can be curative without further treatment. Occasionally, the surgeon will discover that the enlarged testicle has another (non-malignant) cause, but, if so, he or she can simply put it back into the scrotum again and sew up the wound.

Post-operative chemotherapy is likely to be given over a three- to four-month period, generally with four courses of drugs. Details do, of course, vary from centre to centre, but most large hospitals use either cisplatin or carboplatin, together with bleomycin and etoposide (see page 28). The drugs are generally pretty well tolerated, particularly with modern anti-nausea treatments, in marked contrast to the situation in the 1970s, when chemotherapy for testicular tumours was really taking off, but invariably made patients dreadfully ill before (sometimes) curing them.

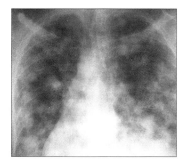

Characteristic chest X-ray of secondary lung deposits from testicular cancer. Patients like these are often still curable because chemotherapy is so effective in this condition.

FOLLOW-UP TREATMENT

Teratoma tumours: If patients have stage 1 (localised) disease, they are nowadays increasingly followed up without further treatment, particularly where the tumour is a teratoma. This policy of surveillance seems increasingly justified and the patient obviously needs careful follow-up with scanning and marker studies.

PAUL'S STORY

Paul, a journalist of 24, was somewhat embarrassed by his swollen testicle. He'd first noticed it a month or so before and he didn't quite know what to do about it. You would have thought he'd have gone to see his doctor straight away, but for some reason it didn't occur to him that this was the sort of thing that you bothered your GP about – after all, he felt so well! But, in the end, he did go. By this time, it was clearly getting bigger and was about twice its previous size. There had been no pain, and, in response to his doctor's questioning, he agreed to check with his mother whether there had been any history of late testicular descent when he was a child.

He went back for the second time, after a week of antibiotics, with the information the doctor had asked for: 'When I was four, I apparently had to have an operation to stitch the testicle into the scrotum.' That just about clinched it. There certainly hadn't been any reduction in testicular size with the antibiotics, and the GP arranged an urgent appointment with the local urologist. Several blood tests and a testicular ultrasound later, it was clear that this must certainly be a malignant testicular tumour. The testicular ultrasound had confirmed that this was a solid, not a cystic, mass.

Paul was admitted to hospital in a state of considerable anxiety. He couldn't quite believe what was happening to him, nor that the surgeon could possibly be right when he assured him that one testicle is all you need. His sense of foreboding was all the stronger when the post-operative scanning tests confirmed evidence of glandular disease in the abdomen, with only a modest fall in the circulating marker levels. Histologically, this had proven to be a mixed testicular teratoma, and the oncologist was blunt: 'You certainly need chemotherapy, you need it now, and it'll almost certainly cure you.'

Five years after the treatment, Paul's wife presented him with a son, and his annual follow-up visits are now more for the hospital's students' and trainees' benefit than his own. With testicular teratomas, patients who have achieved three trouble-free years from diagnosis are virtually always cured, so strictly speaking, they don't need to be all that vigilant.

Seminoma tumours: It's less straightforward with seminoma since these tumours don't make a marker so regular scanning is even more essential. In addition, the traditional treatment with post-operative radiotherapy has been pretty successful in this group, as a result of their quite remarkable sensitivity and responsiveness to radiation therapy. For this reason, only small doses of radiotherapy need be given to the abdominal and pelvic lymph node areas, generally without any long-term disadvantage. The dilemma persists, and a recent interesting proposal is the possibility of using just a single course of single drug post-operative chemotherapy, on the grounds that this may well be enough in patients who already have an excellent prognosis anyway.

prognosis

Life with only one testicle is perfectly OK. There shouldn't be any alteration to sexual potency, since levels of hormone (testosterone) from a single testicle is more than enough. Even where both testes have been involved (it does occasionally happen) and have to be removed, male hormones can be replaced by injection, many patients requiring them approximately every two or three months. These restore the normal levels of testosterone in the majority of cases.

Fertility, however, is another matter. There is a small but significant group of patients with testicular tumours who are sub-fertile right from the outset, even before surgery or chemotherapy. In some patients, the testicular malignancy is even diagnosed this way, the patient coming as part of a couple to an infertility clinic and blissfully unaware of the testicular mass that is present and responsible for his producing insufficient sperm. Chemotherapy certainly reduces the sperm count as well, so much so that sperm storage should always be offered prior to treatment with chemotherapy, though many patients have in the end restoration of adequate sperm counts as time goes by after successful chemotherapy. It is always a great pleasure to be able to throw out the frozen (cryopreserved) sperm samples taken three or four years beforehand, of a man who is not only cured and potent but also evidently capable of fathering a child as well – in the normal way.

Despite all this good news, there is no doubt that the diagnosis and treatment of testicular tumours does produce considerable psychological stress. After all, many of these young patients are just approaching manhood, and there is probably no worse time to be told you've developed a malignant illness, let alone of the testis. Some adolescent boys, aware of a testicular mass, keep it very much to themselves for far too long because of embarrassment or fear; fortunately, they generally turn out to have a benign cause for the mass, such as a dilatation of the spermatic cord or of the blood vessels surrounding it.

As recently as the 1980s, patients with testicular teratomas that had spread up to the abdomen or chest had very little chance of cure, but the outlook has now been revolutionised by the advent of effective chemotherapy. For patients with localised disease, the cure rate is virtually 100%, and even in the more advanced stages, remains above 90% in large specialist centres offering the best in terms of investigation, treatment and supportive care. Although often young and vulnerable, patients with testicular tumours can expect a return to a normal life – one of Britain's most celebrated patients, Bob Champion, even went on to win the Grand National, helping the public towards a recognition that cancer doesn't have to be an inevitable death sentence.

SKIN CANCER

The skin is the body's largest and most accessible organ and is subject to all sorts of potentially harmful influences, including sunlight, so it's no surprise that skin cancers are the most common of all malignancies. Many people are well aware of the rising incidence of skin cancer, unfortunately related to our predilection for sun exposure, together with an enormous increase in visits to sunny holiday destinations abroad, and the serious disruption of the protective ozone layer.

● It has been known for over two centuries that skin cancers can develop as a result of directly applied carcinogens, the earliest example being the observation of Sir Percivall Pott well before 1800 that chimney sweeps often developed cancer of the scrotum because of direct exposure to soot in the chimney flue.

● Other occupational skin cancers were discovered during the last century.

● More recently, it has become apparent that radiation, so often used to cure cancer, can itself produce skin cancers. For example, it used to be common to treat ringworm of the scalp with radiation but this is now totally unacceptable because of the high incidence of cancers developing later on within the irradiated area.

● There is no doubt whatever of the importance of sunlight in the development of skin cancers. Skin cancer develops directly in proportion to the intensity of sunlight, and is far more common in Australia and South Africa, for example, than in Europe. In the UK, most occur on an exposed part of the body, particularly the scalp and face. They are far more common in pale-skinned than non-white races, particularly people with very pale, Celtic colouring.

● Immune suppression is important, too. Patients with transplanted kidneys or other organs, who need long-term immunosuppressive therapy, are probably a hundred times more likely to develop skin cancers.

● In AIDS, one of the most common malignant conditions is Kaposi's sarcoma, generally a multi-focal type of skin malignancy and previously uncommon. In addition, there are one or two inherited disorders in which skin malignancy is more prevalent, including albinism (loss of skin pigment) and Gorlin's syndrome, characterised by multiple skin tumours and skeletal abnormalities. In albinism it is probably the lack of skin pigment to filter out sun rays that leads to high rates of skin cancer.

SKIN CANCER KEY POINTS

Basal cell carcinomas
● Very common, but metastasise very rarely, so no reason to refer urgently.

● Majority are on the face, particularly around the nose and the area where the eyes touch the nose.

Squamous cell carcinomas
● About 9,000 to 10,000 each year in England and Wales.

● Rare in patients aged less than 60 years.

● Most common locations for both sexes are face and back of hands; for men, the scalp and ears, and for women, the lower legs.

Malignant melanomas
● 4,000 cases each year in England and Wales.

● Distribution in men: head and neck 25%, upper limb 17%, trunk 37%, lower limb 21%.

● Distribution in women: head and neck 14%, upper limb 18%, trunk 14%, lower limb 53%.

● Affects all adult age groups.

● Most common locations for women are 50% on lower leg; for men, 33% on back.

Solar ultraviolet (UV) radiation in relation to the Earth and the ozone layer. UVA and UVB radiation pass through the ozone layer and reach the Earth while the more harmful UVC radiation is removed by the ozone layer.

symptoms and diagnosis

Reducing the rapidly rising incidence of skin cancer has become a major health priority. It really is important, when sunbathing or skiing, to provide protection from burning, most particularly in childhood. Although the public are becoming increasingly aware of the dangers, it is hard to see the incidence of skin cancers falling, and education has largely shifted towards early detection of potentially dangerous skin lesions. Any pigmented or crusted area, which becomes painful or starts to blister or bleed, should be taken seriously. Far better to bother the doctor with a trivial skin lesion than to miss a potentially serious one at a stage when it can't be so easily dealt with.

The main types of skin cancer are basal cell and squamous cell carcinoma, melanoma, skin lymphoma and Kaposi's sarcoma. The first two (basal and squamous cell carcinomas) are much the most common, indeed the basal cell carcinoma (often known as a rodent ulcer) accounts for about three-quarters of all cases of skin malignancy in the Western world. Finally, many types of lymphoma (chiefly the non-Hodgkin's variety rather than Hodgkin's disease) can occur in the skin, and these are discussed on pages 153-8.

BASAL CELL CARCINOMAS

These are more common with increasing age and are unusual in anyone aged less than 30 years, apart from the few cases that present as a result of an inherited disorder or early exposure to radiation. They have a very characteristic appearance and invade and destroy the skin locally, without any tendency to metastasise to other parts of the body.

- Usually about 2 to 5 millimetres when diagnosed, they're typically painless but often itchy.
- They often have a rolled 'pearly' edge.
- They don't provoke any local lymph node involvement.
- They are common on the scalp and face, especially around the eyes and nose.
- Occasionally, if neglected, they can grow to a very large size.

APPEARANCE OF BASAL CELL CARCINOMAS

Slowly growing red pearly nodule on skin surface. Later it may break down with crusting and ulcerate.

SQUAMOUS CELL CARCINOMAS

Squamous cell carcinomas of the skin are somewhat more dangerous since they have the capacity to produce local lymphatic invasion with nodal enlargement. They also tend to spread more laterally (sideways) under the skin surface, an important point when considering treatment.
● They are generally caused by sunlight exposure and therefore have a similar distribution – face, scalp, neck, hands and forearms.
● They occasionally occur in areas of previous radiation exposure and if so, are likely to be both clinically and pathologically more aggressive, though the interval between the radiation exposure and the later development of the cancer is generally about 20 years.

> **APPEARANCE OF SQUAMOUS CELL CARCINOMAS**
>
> Slowly growing, non-healing lesions, which become hard when pressed and expand over a period of 1 to 2 months.

MALIGNANT MELANOMAS

Malignant melanoma, arising from pigmented skin cells and the most feared type of skin malignancy, is a different kettle of fish. Much more dangerous than either basal or squamous cell cancers, it has dramatically increased in incidence during the last 50 years (at least 5% per year from 1950 onwards), and is particularly common in Australia, New Zealand and South Africa, where the risk is about ten times as great as in the UK. Again, its incidence increases with age, and it chiefly occurs on sun-exposed areas, far more commonly in whites than blacks, presumably as a result of the effectiveness of pigmented skin in screening out solar ultraviolet light, so important in the causation of the disease.

The trouble is that it can be extremely difficult to diagnose, since all of us have freckles and moles, and we don't on the whole pay them much attention, particularly those on areas of our bodies that we can't easily see. Although it's perfectly possible to keep an eye on these, skin clinics have increasingly recognised the difficulties and become far more accessible
● Any change such as crusting, bleeding, enlargement, blistering or itching, should certainly be taken seriously and shown to the family doctor or local 'walk-in' skin clinic.
● The overwhelming majority of moles on our bodies are completely innocent, and always remain so. However, more than half of all melanomas arise from pre-existing benign naevi (pigmented skin areas), though some clearly do develop at sites of previously normal skin.
● Naevi that change in appearance and develop an irregular edge should be viewed with suspicion, particularly if they increase in thickness, since the most reliable guide to eventual outcome is the depth of the invasion or thickness of the tumour.

> **APPEARANCE OF MALIGNANT MELANOMAS**
>
> *Major signs*
> ● If an existing mole gets larger or a new one is growing.
> ● If the mole has an irregular outline.
> ● If the colours are mixed shades of brown or black.
>
> *Minor signs*
> ● If the mole is bigger than the blunt end of a pencil.
> ● If it is inflamed or has a reddish edge.
> ● If it is bleeding, oozing or crusting.
> ● If it starts to feel different: for example, itching or painful.

KAPOSI'S SARCOMA

Kaposi's sarcoma, originally described just over a hundred years ago, was a very unusual tumour, at least in most of Europe, before the start of the AIDS epidemic in the early 1980s. In Africa, however, it is fairly common (non-AIDS related), accounting for up to 10% of all cancers in

JAMES' AND EDWARD'S STORIES

By a curious coincidence, James and Edward, both 62 years of age and recently retired from the armed forces, met in the waiting room of the skin clinic just over five years ago. They had known each other well in earlier years, but had lost touch.

James was the first to be called in. He had a small, crusted lesion just behind his left ear, about a centimetre across, which had been present for three months. It wasn't pigmented or painful, but it had certainly increased in size and had bled on two or three occasions. A small biopsy was taken there and then, and a week later, the dermatologist explained that this was a squamous cell carcinoma and could be removed surgically or treated by radiotherapy. No glands were enlarged, and there was no evidence of other skin tumours. Somewhat alarmed by the prospect of surgery on his ear, James opted for radiotherapy and came along for treatment as an out-patient on ten occasions over the next month. Six months later at his follow-up visit, his tumour had healed beautifully with no scarring or residual ulceration. Three other small primaries of a very similar nature were diagnosed and treated over the following three years, all at sun-affected sites – he'd served his country for over 30 years, chiefly in India and the Far East, paying little regard to skin coverage. For two years now, there hasn't been any sign of new tumours, and he's certainly cured of all the treated ones.

The dermatologist was much more concerned about Edward's 'little problem', as he described it. Not so little: a 2-centimetre, heavily pigmented (almost black), irregularly shaped tumour over his left thigh, clearly raised above the surrounding skin, with a slightly pale centre and a reddened flare around it. The dermatologist thought he could feel one or two glands present in the left groin: Edward's physical condition was otherwise unremarkable. A small biopsy confirmed the fears of the dermatologist that this was a nodular malignant melanoma – quite a thick one. He didn't much like the feel of the glands in the groin either, and conveyed these fears to the surgeon, who agreed to see Edward as a matter of urgency.

The surgeon recommended wide excision of the primary tumour, with skin grafting, together with the removal of glands in the groin, making it clear to Edward that this was quite a substantial procedure requiring a week or two in hospital. Although all went well, Edward soon realised how serious his condition was when the report from the pathology lab confirmed that melanoma cells had been found in the glandular areas as well as the apparently normal skin surrounding the obvious primary site.

He healed up well and had no further problems during the first nine months of follow-up, but when he went to the hospital for a routine follow-up visit, he fell as he stood up from his chair. Reluctantly, he admitted to having been dizzy for over a fortnight, with two falls. Later that day an urgent CT brain scan confirmed that he had a small but critically sited secondary deposit in the cerebellum, at the back of the brain, which was clearly a metastasis from the melanoma. Since there didn't seem to be any further deposits, and he was otherwise clear, the brain surgeon saw him, and they operated the following week. Once again, the pathology lab confirmed that this was indeed a melanoma secondary, and he underwent radiotherapy treatment to the brain, which was done on an out-patient basis over a two-week period.

Somewhat to everyone's surprise, it was 18 months before anything further went wrong. In the meantime, Edward enjoyed an excellent quality of life and travelled to California to see his grandchildren. At the end of that time, though, he appeared in the out-patient's clinic, again quite obviously unwell. The complaints were of shortness of breath and increasing weakness, and a chest X-ray showed widespread secondary tumours. Edward refused chemotherapy and requested transfer to the local hospice. He had considerable family and professional support, and responded to several of the palliative measures that were still possible, even though cure was clearly out of the question.

parts of East Africa. The European form is a disease of immunosuppression, occurring in AIDS patients and those with renal transplants. In patients with transplants the immune suppression (which allows the tumour to develop) can be reversed if the immune-reductive drugs are discontinued, whereas in AIDS, of course, this is not possible.

● The lesions look pigmented, often very dark, with nodules typically appearing on the leg or foot, often growing rather slowly.

● Ulceration may occur, or they may become confluent.

● In AIDS, the disease often involves lymph node and other sites, notably the lining of the mouth, developing faster than non-AIDS cases.

BASAL CELL CARCINOMAS

They are almost always curable. Surgery and radiotherapy both work well, but there is evidence that surgery may be slightly more effective on the face. The treatment recommendation often depends on the preference of the dermatologist and the quality of local services. Radiotherapy has the advantage that the patient avoids an operation and loss of local tissues, though in truth, most such operations are small and very straightforward, generally under local anaesthesia. Although radiotherapy takes longer (typically two to three weeks of treatment, though not necessarily every day) it can be preferable, for example around the eyes, where surgery may cause damage. With large rodent ulcers, wider surgery and skin grafting is sometimes necessary.

SQUAMOUS CELL CARCINOMAS

Treatment by surgery or radiotherapy is generally very effective, though a wider area has to be excised (or irradiated) than in the case of basal cell carcinomas, because of the pathological characteristics of these tumours, particularly their greater degree of lateral spread. Patients with lymph node involvement are generally treated by surgery, both for the primary tumour and the nodal metastases. Again, skin grafting may sometimes be necessary and the cosmetic results are usually very good.

MALIGNANT MELANOMAS

Surgery: If the skin biopsy does confirm a malignant melanoma, then surgical excision is essential – the most important form of treatment. This should be undertaken by a specialist with particular experience; plastic surgeons often have a special expertise since wide surgical excision has traditionally been recommended, and for adequate skin coverage of the defect this will often require grafting. This is recommended because of the wide, intradermal infiltration that may occur, though recent reports suggest that surgery can perhaps be rather more conservative than was traditionally recommended.

Malignant melanomas often spread by nodal involvement, usually into local or regional areas, and some surgeons recommend surgery and node removal at these sites as well. The general view, however, is that

treatment

ESTABLISHED ASSOCIATIONS BETWEEN SUNLIGHT AND MELANOMA

● The incidence of melanoma varies with latitude. For populations with the same skin colour, the nearer the equator, the higher the incidence.

● Studies of emigrants to Australia and New Zealand show that those who arrive over the age of 15 have a lower incidence than those born in these sunny countries.
Thus early childhood sun exposure is important.

● The incidence is 1 to 12 times higher in white-skinned races who have little protective melanin pigment by comparison with black-skinned races living the same lifestyle.

● Among white-skinned individuals, those with particularly fair skin that burns easily and tans poorly are at most risk.

● Individual sun exposure habits affect the risk.

● Case control studies show severe sunburn to be a risk factor.

this confers no survival benefit, apart from patients in whom node metastases are already present at the time of initial diagnosis (usually a very adverse feature), but can at least be surgically removed.

For localised lesions less than 1.5 millimetres thick, the outcome following surgical resection is, on the whole, pretty good; in fact, the really superficial ones, less than 0.75 millimetres, rarely spread beyond the primary site, and surgery is usually curative.

Radiotherapy: This has a role in the management of melanoma, but is generally used for controlling secondary tumours, particularly in bone or brain, where it remains the best form of treatment.

Chemotherapy: Although chemotherapy is not yet very effective for melanoma, there are cases on record where substantial tumour shrinkage has taken place. Australian specialists, who see far more melanoma than British specialists do, have claimed the occasional cure, even with patients who have disseminated disease.

Immunotherapy: Treatment with BCG (see page 214), or even denatured melanoma cells, has produced local responses in patients with recurrent skin lesions or lymph node involvement, though most of the responses are brief. Interferon is also increasingly used in melanoma, and has been claimed to extend the recurrence-free interval following primary surgery. There are also reports of very occasional spontaneous regression in melanoma, or shrinkage of established disease during a pregnancy, raising the possibility of either an active immune benefit or a clinically valuable degree of hormone sensitivity; as is often the case, however, when anecdote turns into clinical trial, the overall results from a larger number of patients look less encouraging than we had initially hoped.

KAPOSI'S SARCOMA

Most Kaposi lesions respond well to radiotherapy, and a single treatment is often sufficient, though many AIDS patients require multiple areas of treatment. Chemotherapy can also be useful, but patients with AIDS are at risk of so many other problems, both infectious and malignant, that survival is often compromised by other complications.

prognosis

In conclusion, skin cancers are common, relatively easy to spot, and, to a large extent, preventable by a sensible approach to sunlight exposure. The majority are easily curable by surgery or radiotherapy and pose little threat. On the other hand, malignant melanoma is a far more serious diagnosis and must be recognised and treated as early as possible. Worrying pigmented lesions should always be looked at by a family doctor, in the first instance, or skin clinic. If necessary, a biopsy can then be performed and treatment recommended as appropriate.

OTHER CANCERS

HEAD AND NECK CANCERS

These tumours are, fortunately, not very common: about 4% of all cancer diagnosed in the UK each year. They are extremely important, though, posing exceptional problems of management and rehabilitation, since they can be highly visible and sometimes disfiguring. Surgical treatment can also lead to loss of function (speech, swallowing, etc.) or to permanent changes of appearance.

causes

Cancers of the larynx (voice apparatus), pharynx (throat), oral cavity (mouth, including tongue, palate, jaw, etc.) and nasal region are included in this group. Although fairly uncommon in the UK, they are much more prevalent in other parts of the world.

● In southern China and Hong Kong, for example, tumours at the back of the nose (nasopharynx) are the most common of all cancers, possibly related to a diet that is high in preserved or pickled foods and salted fish, which might contain high concentrations of carcinogens.

● In parts of India, where chewing tobacco and betel nut is widely practised, tumours of the oral cavity (particularly the cheek area) are commonplace because of the direct placement (sometimes all day) of a tobacco-containing pouch against the cheek lining.

● In the West, though, the most common cause of many of these tumours (notably oral cavity and parts of the throat) is a high intake of alcohol combined with heavy smoking, a situation in which the risk is increased by about 20 times, in comparison with the normal population.

● Cancer of the larynx, a tumour clearly related to cigarette smoking, has no definite link with alcohol.

Overall, these cancers are more common in men, and the past 30 years have seen a fall in incidence due to improvements in dental and oral hygiene, coupled with reduction in cigarette and alcohol intake, though in parts of Europe the number of cases (particularly of oral cancer) is starting to rise again as a result of increasing alcohol consumption. At other sites, notably the lip, there has been a reduction in incidence, probably due to the decreasing popularity of pipe smoking, previously responsible for many cases.

HEAD AND NECK CANCERS KEY POINTS
Incidence: 7,000 cases each year in England and Wales.
Risk factors: ● Smoking (90%)   ● Tobacco chewing habits   ● Alcohol   ● Poor diet   ● Social deprivation   ● Older age

symptoms and diagnosis

Pathologically, these cancerous cells are typical squamous carcinomas, i.e. tumours that arise from the surface lining (see page 28). They tend to ulcerate early, at least when situated in the mouth.

● A common symptom is of a persistent, non-healing ulcer recognised as potentially malignant by the family doctor or dentist.

MOST COMMON SYMPTOMS OF HEAD AND NECK CANCERS

Larynx
Hoarseness 80-90%
Pain on swallowing 30-40%
Dysphagia 30%

Pharynx
Lump in the neck 80-90%
Nasal obstruction 60%
Deafness 50%
Post-nasal discharge 40-50%

Oral cavity
Ulceration/visible lesion 80%
Pain 60%
Lump in the neck 20-40%

Nasal cavity
Obstruction/congestion 80-90%
Bleeding 70-80%

● **Tumours in the oral cavity** are sometimes detected early, though some sites are notoriously easily missed, notably an ulcer situated in the floor of the mouth, beneath the tongue.

● **In cancer of the larynx**, hoarseness of the voice is much the most common symptom. Any complaint of hoarseness by a patient that is greater than three weeks' duration should be taken seriously and referred to an ear, nose and throat (ENT) specialist for examination of the vocal cords, since early laryngeal cancer is readily detected and effectively treated. If left, however, cure may be impossible without removal of the larynx (laryngectomy) and permanent loss of the natural speaking voice.

● **In the pharynx**, the most common symptoms are difficulty with swallowing, since the tumour may obstruct the passage of food; or of nasal stuffiness and discharge, if the tumour is situated in the upper part of the pharynx, behind the nose.
● Surprisingly, many of these tumours are painless, though they may cause other symptoms due to their proximity to the base of the skull, and the vulnerability of the nervous pathways coursing downwards at that level.
● Many head and neck cancers spread to the lymph glands of the neck, and it isn't at all uncommon for patients to have a swollen gland or lymph node in the neck but without any other recognisable effect or symptom.
● A tumour might well be visibly detectable to an expert, possibly arising from a relatively inaccessible site, such as the back end of the upper pharynx or tonsil, though the truth, of course, is that enlarged glands in the neck are much more likely due to infections or other minor conditions, either self-limiting or quickly and easily brought under control with a course of antibiotics.
● If the lymph node is really large, however, cancer becomes a much more likely cause.

Apart from glandular spread, head and neck tumours, as a group, don't on the whole disseminate to other parts of the body. Achieving permanent control of the primary site – including, of course, the neck glands – is usually tantamount to a cure. The main exception to this rule is in patients with nasopharyngeal cancers, a group which behave rather differently from the others, with a different causation and pattern of spread. They have a typical pattern of early invasion of lymph nodes in the neck and a greater propensity for widespread involvement of distant sites of the body. Unlike other head and neck primary sites, radical surgery plays little or no part in their management.

Clinical staging is extremely important. Early tumours carry a much better outlook than more advanced ones, and if there is no evidence of lymph node involvement, they do on the whole have a relatively good

SURGERY, RADIOTHERAPY OR BOTH?

The consequences of treatment by radiotherapy or surgery may well govern the choice of which method to recommend. The careful consideration and choice of treatment, together with a full explanation to the patient, is the kind of issue that can only be settled in a combined head-and-neck oncology clinic, case by case, and the chosen treatment for one patient may be inappropriate for another.

With cancers of the mouth and mid-pharynx area, radiotherapy may certainly cure, but probably at the cost of a dry mouth and some degree of long-term oral discomfort. There is no easy way of relieving these symptoms, but many patients manage pretty well by keeping a small bottle of water to sip throughout the day or by using an artificial saliva aerosol spray.

Surgical treatment, on the other hand, can lead to permanent loss of tissue, which may not always be easy to reconstruct, despite many attempts at functional repair. An honest discussion of these issues before treatment is the best means of ensuring a satisfied patient afterwards.

When patients do have enlarged glands in the neck, it is possible to remove them surgically using an operation that has certainly stood the test of time, the radical neck node dissection. This can often be achieved without serious, long-term consequences and with a very acceptable cosmetic result. The alternative is to irradiate the whole of the neck, and undertake such surgery only if radiotherapy fails to control the glandular involvement. Most patients find surgery to the neck a less troublesome operation than surgery at the primary site.

As far as surgical reconstruction is concerned, there seems no limit to the ingenuity of plastic surgeons, who nowadays seem to be able to perform reconstuctions that wouldn't have been contemplated not so long ago. Before a final treatment decision is taken, the best means of evaluation is by an experienced team of surgeons and radiotherapists working together, with any implications being fully discussed with the patient at the appropriate moment.

prognosis. It is much more difficult to cure patients with obvious malignant lymph node infiltration in the neck. Visible, accessible tumours may be easy to stage, even without an anaesthetic, but cancers situated at deeper sites – for example, larynx and nasopharynx – will need full inspection under anaesthetic.

Scanning is important since it may detect an otherwise impalpable degree of neck node involvement or give additional information as to the true extent of the primary tumour. Either or both of these features may determine the operability of the cancer.

treatment

More than any other tumour types, cancers of the head and neck are reminders that cancer is not a single disease but a group of disorders, each case bearing its own characteristics of site, local involvement, extension to lymph nodes and so on. Each site requires special consideration, and although it's possible to make general recommendations about treatment, a degree of individualisation is often necessary for the best management approach. The surgeon and radiotherapist should work closely together, together with dental and prosthetic staff, speech therapists, experts in nutrition and clinical nurse specialists, seeing patients before final treatment decisions are made. It's also an area where rapid changes of management have occurred over the past ten years, with an increasing emphasis now on conservation and reconstructive surgery to minimise the damaging effects of the tumour itself and the treatments on offer.

LARYNGEAL CANCER

Cancer of the larynx is the most common of the head and neck cancers encountered in the UK, far more commonly occurring in men (80%) than women. It is much more prevalent in smokers, occurring chiefly between the ages of 50 and 75, and the most common site is the vocal cord itself, rather than the other parts of the larynx. Although hoarseness is by far the most common complaint, laryngeal cancers can also cause pain or interfere with the swallowing mechanism. Localised tumours are confined to the free edge of the vocal cord, whereas more advanced ones can invade into the cartilaginous supporting structure of the larynx, paralysing the vocal cord completely.

Radiotherapy: Treatment of early cases by radiotherapy is usually highly successful; indeed, one of the greatest successes of radiation therapy is in the very high cure rate (over 90%) of these tumours, without the need for any surgery whatever, generally with full restoration of the voice. The more advanced the laryngeal tumour, the harder this is to achieve, but even cases with paralysis of the vocal cord can sometimes be cured by radiotherapy, though restoration of the voice would not be so good.

As with many cancers, radiotherapy approaches vary considerably, and there is little to choose between a three-week course of treatment, as typically recommended at large centres in the North of England, and a six-week course of treatment, more usually recommended in London and the south. Before the treatment starts, an immobilisation shell is routinely constructed by radiographers to keep the patient completely still on the treatment couch throughout the radiotherapy treatment sessions, since precision is so important in this type of work. The fewer breaks in treatment, the better, so it's extremely important that patients realise the importance of sticking to the recommended treatment plan, and not (as does quite often happen) waltzing off for a day or two's break here and there.

On the whole, side-effects of radiotherapy for laryngeal cancer are fairly well tolerated, though some patients complain of discomfort in the neck area, generally short lived, or an increase in their hoarseness, before recovery starts.

Surgery: 'Salvage' laryngectomy (removal of the larynx with permanent loss of the natural voice) may be necessary if radiotherapy is unsuc-

FRANK'S STORY

Frank had always been a loner. When he first went to his oncology specialist he was 54, had had a series of building and labouring jobs, was separated from his wife, whom he hadn't seen for 25 years, and spent most of his evenings at the pub. He'd been on about 40 cigarettes and half a dozen lagers a day since his early twenties.

His voice had been husky for two months – he had thought this was because of his smoking. Eventually, he'd turned up at casualty and they'd called the ENT registrar, who looked at the vocal cords, saw one was paralysed and realised that there was probably a tumour lurking about. A few days later, Frank's consultant confirmed a laryngeal cancer and decided that radiotherapy would be the best approach, offering at least the possibility of avoiding a laryngectomy. He was treated within a clinical trial, comparing radiotherapy alone with radiotherapy plus chemotherapy: he was allocated treatment with radiotherapy alone.

Frank found the treatment quite tough; but although his radiation reaction settled quickly, the hoarseness did not improve, and, two months after completion of the radiotherapy, a further examination and biopsy by the ENT consultant confirmed that the tumour had not completely gone. Laryngectomy was therefore inevitable, and, realising that this was the only means of saving his life, Frank agreed.

The operation went well, and the surgeon didn't feel that the previous radiotherapy had made it more difficult. Pre-operatively, Frank received excellent counselling from the surgical team, the speech therapist who would be looking after him and from a laryngectomy patient who had gone through the same thing almost a decade before. He was in hospital for three weeks, and, despite his best efforts at producing oesophageal speech by swallowing air and expelling it upwards, he never quite got the hang of it. A few months later, a speech valve was inserted in his neck.

Frank has come out of it all pretty well, and is a faithful attender at his follow-up visits and speech therapy sessions. He's stopped smoking altogether now, but has found it much more difficult to stop drinking. His biggest frustration is not being able to make himself heard at the bar, but, as he pointed out, 'I just have to get the others to buy drinks for me.'

cessful. Surgeons sometimes express misgivings about operating on patients who have previously received radiotherapy, but most patients seem to get through this type of surgery very well, despite the previous radiotherapy. There is little disadvantage in attempting a non-surgical cure apart from cases where the laryngeal obstruction or bulk of tumour is so great that early surgery is mandatory.

Chemotherapy: It looks pretty clear that, as with squamous cell cancers at many other sites of the body, the use of chemotherapy improves the outlook of patients with laryngeal cancer, at least from the point of view of freedom from relapse. This is particularly important in head and neck sites such as the larynx, since the consequences of failure are so damaging, having to resort to permanent laryngectomy or other major surgical procedures. The most effective chemotherapy protocols are those that are given simultaneously, or 'synchronously', with radical radiation therapy.

PHARYNGEAL CANCER

Cancers of the pharynx are a more difficult group. Cure is less commonly achieved than with cancer of the larynx, particularly in patients with cancers situated in the uppermost part, behind the nose, or lowest part of the pharynx. The risk of early lymph node spread is much higher with pharyngeal than laryngeal tumours, greatly reducing the probability of control by radiotherapy with or without surgery.

For nasopharyngeal cancers, the radiotherapy treatment area has to be very substantial to cover the potential lymph node sites on both sides of the neck. Fortunately, facial skin is so well supplied by blood vessels that recovery from radiotherapy is usually excellent, even where the original skin reaction has been severe.

For tumours lower down the pharynx, surgery may have more of a part to play, though some centres rely on radiotherapy, with or without chemotherapy. The high dosage of radiotherapy necessary for cure may result in a very brisk, and sometimes painful, degree of inflammation at the back of the throat and mouth, and assisted feeding by a fine-bore stomach tube is often necessary – it can make all the difference between a well-nourished patient or a totally demoralised one. It is very important that the patient does not lose weight during what can be an extremely tough course of treatment. The involvement of a dietician is important to maintain nutritional input.

CANCER OF THE ORAL CAVITY

In the oral cavity, both surgery and radiotherapy can be highly effective. Because of the accessibility of many of these tumours, radiotherapy with radioactive implants is quite often recommended, for example with cancers of the tongue, palate or lip, since this treatment offers a high radiation dose to the tumour itself, with a rapid fall-off in the dose to other sites. This can be used either by itself or together with external beam irradiation, and is often very successful.

Surgery, too, can be excellent, but with the potential disadvantage of loss of important areas of functional tissue. For example, even small tumours at the side or edge of the tongue may require removal of half of the tongue for clearance, a fairly substantial operative procedure. On the other hand, surgical reconstruction has dramatically improved over the past 20 years. It is now possible to recreate large portions of the lining of the mouth, the upper part of the gullet and other important sites, such that surgical resection of a primary cancer can often be achieved with a reasonably acceptable functional result – and without the permanent dry mouth that radiotherapy can sometimes cause.

NOSE AND LIP CANCERS

Cancers of the nose and lips require a great deal of care, since disfigurement is obviously to be avoided at all costs, if at all possible. Once again, the treatment choice generally lies between surgery and radiotherapy, and there can sometimes be little to choose between them. Radiotherapy may have the edge as far as appearance and function are concerned, though for large tumours, surgical resection and early reconstruction may be preferable. What the patient needs is not only a good cosmetic appearance, but the certainty that his or her mouth will subsequently close properly, so that food can be chewed and swallowed without embarrassing spillage.

THYROID CANCER

Thyroid cancer, a highly specialist area, is a very variable group of disorders, some of which have a remarkably high cure rate. They mostly occur in young women, and can be treated very effectively by surgical removal of the thyroid and, where necessary, the use of radioactive iodine. For diagnosis, ultrasound of the neck, isotope uptake scans, computer tomography (CT) or magnetic resonance imaging (MRI) scanning and biopsy of suspicious nodules are all important.

Radioactive iodine: This treatment depends on the unique ability of the thyroid gland to take up iodine. If radioactive iodine is deliberately given, in the form of capsules swallowed by mouth, then the gland will absorb it, becoming sufficiently radioactive that any residual cancer cells within it are destroyed.

The same technique can also be used for secondary deposits of thyroid cancer at other parts of the body, once the main thyroid gland has been 'ablated' by surgery and the first radioactive dose. The radioactive iodine then permits a highly desirable 'self-destruct' of the secondary deposits, with the consequence that thyroid cancer is one of the few human cancers to be curable even when the tumour has spread beyond the primary site.

MRS PATEL'S STORY

Originally from Bangladesh, Mrs Patel had been in England for 20 years. She'd brought up her four children almost single-handedly since her husband, Haresh, had had a severe stroke only a few years after they had arrived.

She first saw her specialist with a note from the Department of Oral Surgery. They had confirmed her dentist's suspicions of a malignant ulcer involving the floor of the mouth and under-surface of the tongue – too extensive, they felt, for surgical removal. Her daughter was with her and, as is so often the case, acted as interpreter. She wasn't keen on conveying the specialist's thoughts too accurately, since she was anxious to protect her mother from too much bad news all at once. 'But I need to know that she realises the true position,' he said. 'Leave it to me,' she said, 'I'll make sure she understands what she needs to.'

Early during the third week of the radiotherapy, about half way through the total course, Mrs Patel developed a fierce radiation reaction. Neither she nor her daughter were keen for her to come into hospital, but by the fourth week, it was obvious that she would have to, in order to be fed properly. The family's chief concern was centred on who would run the shop. 'Maybe we could ask Daddy's friend Parviz,' said the daughter.

Fate took a hand. Parviz did well, business boomed, a dowry was found. At the six-month follow-up visit, Mrs Patel's daughter smiled shyly as she told her mother's specialist of her forthcoming wedding.

Although Mrs Patel still complained of a painful, dry mouth, she was reassured that there was no evidence of residual cancer, and the artificial saliva spray proved quite helpful. She took it all with philosophical calm. 'Mummy says to tell you that she wouldn't have married me so well if she hadn't got ill and agreed to Parviz's coming into the shop like that.' Her specialist's Bengali wasn't up to much, but they all beamed at each other as she left the clinic, and he made them promise to send a selection of wedding photographs.

Surgery: Thyroid cancers in young people (often collectively termed 'well-differentiated' cancers, in view of their favourable appearance under the microscope) are generally curable by surgery with or without radioactive iodine. The typical type of tumour in patients over the age of 50 is much more difficult to deal with, however, since the tumours tend not to take up iodine (and therefore its radioactive counterpart) so readily as with younger patients. Nonetheless, surgical removal and external irradiation can be extremely valuable, though the overall results aren't nearly so good.

Thyroid supplements: In the long term, virtually all patients treated for cancer of the thyroid will need to take thyroid supplements (thyroxine tablets) for the rest of their life, in order not to develop thyroid under-activity. This is generally a very small price to pay for a highly acceptable method of treatment with an excellent prospect for cure, at least in the younger age group.

Medullary carcinoma of the thyroid: In the case of this particular type of tumour, there is an important association with other tumour types, including benign overgrowth of the adrenal glands (small glands situated close to the kidneys that produce adrenaline and other bioactive substances) and parathyroid enlargement (these glands sit very close to the thyroid and help control calcium metabolism). These syndromes of so-called 'multiple endocrine neoplasia' are often familial, though, curiously, it is generally only the thyroid tumour that is genuinely malignant.

In patients diagnosed with medullary carcinoma, it is extremely important to screen other family members in case they are affected as well. Fortunately, this is generally achieved quite easily by means of checking their blood for a tumour-marker substance – calcitonin – which is usually elevated and easily detected in the bloodstream in patients likely to develop the tumour. Calcitonin levels can also be used to monitor the effect of the treatment.

OTHER HEAD AND NECK CANCERS

Other, rarer tumours of head and neck sites include cancers of the salivary glands, eye and orbit. Most tumours of the salivary glands are benign and dealt with by surgery alone, but in the rare cases of malignant salivary tumours, a combined approach, using surgery and radiotherapy, is generally recommended.

Unfortunately, the facial nerve, which controls the facial muscles, runs right through the middle of the largest salivary gland (which happens to be the most common to be affected by cancer) and permanent paralysis of the facial muscles can be a consequence either of the tumour itself, if it has eroded through the nerve, or of the treatment used to control it.

New techniques are constantly being tried, to attempt a repair of the nerve and provide facial movement again, but the results of these nerve engraftment procedures are still rather uncertain, and plastic surgery to improve the appearance of the drooping side of the face is often the best that can be recommended at present.

Tumours of the orbit, the bony structure encasing the eye, and of the eye itself, are very specialist areas where radiotherapy is generally the most valuable approach, but surgery may also be necessary.

prognosis

Very careful follow-up is essential for head and neck cancers, with monthly visits during the first year of follow-up, and only a gradual easing of the appointments after that. In general, the patient is considered to be cured if, after three years, there has been no evidence of recurrence of the disease.

If the cancer does recur, it is often possible, as described on pages 139-40, to undertake a salvage surgical procedure or, in the case of patients who have not previously received radiotherapy, offer this form of treatment. If the patient is fit and well, it is important not to give up hope at this stage, since head and neck cancers do not generally spread beyond the neck area. Tumour control at the primary site may result in cure, even if a second attempt, for example using 'salvage' surgery, is necessary.

REHABILITATION

As well as careful follow-up, skilled rehabilitation plays an extremely important part in management. Patients may have to learn new techniques for speech and swallowing, or may have to cope with a permanent external prosthesis if there has been surgical disfigurement to a visible part of the face, for example in the case of cancers of the nose or cheek. In the case of patients trying to cope with a laryngectomy, many can be taught by speech therapists to produce a type of speech with reasonable volume and intelligibility, which relies on the swallowing of air, and its expulsion up through the gullet. The resulting 'oesophageal' speech may sound a bit different, but is often highly effective, particularly in extrovert and well-motivated people who can accompany it with theatrical gestures! One alternative that is gaining in popularity is the use of the speech prosthesis, using a small valve inserted into the pharynx area, which some patients can use very effectively after only a little practice.

For patients who have undergone operations to the pharynx, rehabilitation of swallowing is often a difficult and frustrating task. It is one thing to cure the cancer, quite another to provide an adequate swallowing mechanism. One real advantage of radiotherapy over surgery for these tumours is the lesser degree of swallowing difficulty that patients enjoy if surgery can be avoided.

SOFT-TISSUE SARCOMAS

causes

Sarcomas are a curious and unusual group of cancers. Unlike the much more common carcinomas, which are essentially malignant processes involving the lining (as, for example, in the bowel), covering surface (for example, the skin) or glandular structures (for example, breast, thyroid or pancreas), the sarcomas are malignant disorders of the parts in between, so to speak – muscular structures, fat, connecting tissue and bone. Not surprisingly, there is a tremendous variety, including both soft-tissue (covered on these pages) and pathologically distinct primary bone tumours (discussed separately overleaf on page 144). They should not be confused with the secondary deposits in bone which occur in so many cancers and very much more commonly than any of the primary bone malignancies.

Almost nothing is known of their cause, though a few families with a genetic disorder predisposing to sarcomas have been identified. Radiation, too, can undoubtedly cause these tumours, though fortunately, only rarely. For example, there is very well-documented evidence of primary bone tumours developing in the jaws of radium dial workers, mostly young women, whose job was to paint the radium on to watch faces in order to make them luminous. Little was known of the hazard of radium ingestion, and their habit was to suck the tip of their brush to a fine point to enable them to perform the task well. There are appalling cases on record as a result of the very high local doses of radium deposited in the jaws, leading to painful erosion and decay of the bone, combined with the development of osteosarcoma, one of the major varieties of primary malignant bone tumour. In a tiny minority of patients given therapeutic irradiation, a sarcoma of bone, cartilage or soft tissues can develop (usually 10 to 20 years later) within the treated area; fortunately, the risk of this is remote, compared with the many benefits of radiation therapy for malignant disease.

SOFT-TISSUE SARCOMA KEY POINTS

Incidence:
About 1,000 cases each year in the UK.

Age:
Can occur at any age, although it is more common over 30 years.

• Most soft tissue masses are benign (only 1 in 200 are malignant).

• Lumps that are superficial and painless and less than 5cm and static in size are extremely unlikely to be malignant.

---

symptoms and diagnosis

Typically, the patient with a soft-tissue sarcoma complains of a painless lump, most frequently on the trunk, neck, back or limb. Most lumps that people notice on their bodies are entirely benign – a bruise, perhaps (the history of trauma is often, curiously, not recalled); a lipoma, often referred to as a 'fatty lump' and of no sinister significance at all; or various types of innocent cyst or some other benign skin appendage or fluid sac (bursa), commonly occurring at or near a joint. 'Tennis elbow' is a good example of one of these benign conditions. The obviously fluid-filled ones are virtually always benign, but firm (particularly very firm) lumps should be taken seriously, and a biopsy may be necessary.

• As far as symptoms are concerned, that is usually more or less all there is to it, although in some types of soft-tissue sarcoma there can also be glandular involvement of the lymph node group that drains the affected area – the groin, for example, in the case of a mass on the thigh, or the armpit in the case of many trunk or upper limb tumours.

● Soft-tissue sarcomas can occur at any age, and there is certainly a small peak in incidence, both for soft-tissue and bone sarcomas, around the age of 20, after which the frequency falls again, rising again around the age of 60 years. In the soft-tissue group, there are at least half a dozen major varieties, depending on the precise type of tissue from which they originate; although most soft-tissue lumps are completely benign, the malignant group have a great capacity for spread, chiefly by lymph node involvement and also the blood-borne route, typically to the lungs. Other important, potential sites include the liver, bone marrow and brain.

In suspicious cases, a biopsy is essential to confirm or exclude the diagnosis; it is important for the pathologist to specify which particular type of soft-tissue sarcoma it is – they all have long names and behave slightly differently from each other. The major types include:

● Leiomyosarcoma, originating from smooth muscle cells, such as the wall of the female uterus (womb).

● Rhabdomyosarcoma, from a striped muscle primary site, such as thigh, calf or forearm.

● Liposarcoma, from a fatty primary site.

MOST COMMON SYMPTOMS OF SOFT-TISSUE SARCOMAS
Soft tissue mass that is larger than 5cm
Painful
Increasing in size
Deep to fascia
Recurrence after previous excision

treatment

The most important of treatments is adequate surgical removal, with the emphasis on wide excision and generous margins of apparently normal tissue wherever possible. In the case of muscular primaries, the whole muscle must be removed if possible (as, for example, in the uterus, a relatively common primary site for leiomyosarcoma), or at least the muscular compartment from which the tumour has arisen. Surgical clearance may have to be substantial, and ideally the surgeon should not encounter the tumour during the operation to avoid spillage of tumour contents. The next step in treatment should be local irradiation of the whole area to as high a dose as possible, since these tumours are not as radio-sensitive as typical carcinomas, and therefore require a higher local dose for adequate control. This conservative method of treatment has, however, largely replaced (though not quite completely) the traditional surgical approach of limb amputation for a soft-tissue sarcoma of the extremity; in the past, this was all that could be offered.

Opinions are divided as to whether patients should then be given prophylactic (or adjuvant) chemotherapy, but, on the whole, despite many years of thorough research, this approach is not clearly established as beneficial, and should probably be recommended only as part of a clinical trial. On the other hand, if patients do relapse at a distant site such as the lung, there is really no active alternative, apart from the unusual case where relapse is late and confined to a single site which could be surgically removable (such as a single or perhaps a couple of secondary deposits in the lung). Generally speaking, it is either

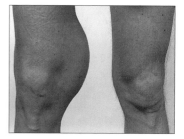

Characteristic appearance of a mass or swelling in the soft tissues – a highly malignant sarcoma arising from the tissues around the knee. This particular patient only sought medical advice when he was unable to put on his trousers. The tumour proved to be a liposarcoma (see text).

chemotherapy or nothing – and the chemotherapy may well be worth-while, particularly in a young, fit patient with measurable disease, which can be closely watched for response. Although a reasonable approach under the circumstances, treatment in this setting will be given to try to produce a lengthy period of control rather than, in all honesty, a real expectation of long-term survival or cure.

MALIGNANT BONE TUMOURS

symptoms and diagnosis

In the case of primary malignant bone tumours, the situation is differ-ent to soft-tissue sarcomas (see previous pages) in several important respects. The two most common types of tumour, both chiefly tumours of adolescence and young adults, are osteosarcoma and Ewing's tumour – pathologically quiet distinct from each other.

OSTEOSARCOMA

Osteosarcoma is the more common and accounts for about a third of all malignant bone tumours, though their rarity is illustrated by the fact that there are fewer than 200 new cases in Britain each year. The tumour arises directly from the bone, typically in an adolescent (boys rather more commonly than girls), producing a very firm mass. The most common site is around the knee, accounting for about two-thirds of all cases. Many give a history of trauma, but the conventional medical view is that the trauma has nothing to do with causation per se, but more likely brought it to medical attention. For further information on the causes of bone tumours see soft-tissue sarcomas on page 142. The mass itself, though always very firm, is often pain free, though not always.

EWING'S TUMOUR

The pathology under the microscope is different to that of osteosar-coma and the sites more variable, with about half of all cases occurring in the lower limb, though not necessarily clustered around the knee.

DIAGNOSIS

It is often possible to make a fairly secure diagnosis after the X-ray, even before surgical biopsy, since the appearances of these two bone tumours are often very characteristic (and different from each other) to an experienced bone radiologist. In fact, it is worth stating firmly that these tumours are so rare that they should always, if at all possible, be handled by specialist panels consisting not only of clinicians (orthopaedic surgeons and oncologists), but also pathologists and diag-nostic radiologists with a particular interest in the subject. Even the site and nature of the surgical biopsy is extremely important, since getting this wrong can sometimes spell disaster or, if not quite that, then unnecessary difficulty in confirming the diagnosis. In older patients, tumours of the cartilage, rather than the bone itself, are more common.

BONE TUMOUR KEY POINTS

Incidence:
About 400 cases each year
in the UK.

Age:
Most common in adolescence.

**MOST COMMON SYMPTOMS
OF BONE TUMOURS**

Pain, which is typically
non-mechanical, waking the patient
at night

Soft tissue mass that is larger
than 5cm

Painful

Increasing in size

Deep to fascia

Recurrence after previous excision

FIONA'S STORY

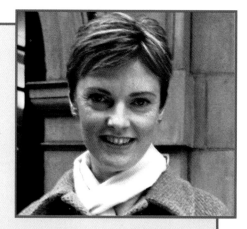

Fiona is a 34-year-old primary school teacher who lives in south-west London. In November 1999, she noticed her leg would occasionally ache in the mornings – but because she was attending a gym she thought it was just that she was over-exercising and left it but by the next March she noticed her leg had become slightly swollen. It wasn't until June that she decided to seek advice from her GP.

Fiona was sent to have an X-ray of her leg and when she went back for the results her GP informed her that there was a tumour and as it was so large it was probably a malignant bone tumour. Fiona recalls, 'That was probably the worst moment ever, after that nothing is as bad as being told in the first place.' Two days later she saw a specialist and three days after that she was admitted to hospital. During this period Fiona said it preyed on her mind as to why she hadn't got advice earlier and to begin with she blamed herself.

Fiona was to have a biopsy and it wasn't until the tissue was examined that there would be a definitive diagnosis. Fiona had had a lot of information to take on board and realised that although the surgeons do try to do limb-sparing operations there was a possibility that she might have to have her leg removed. However, the orthopaedic surgeon who was a specialist in bone tumours warned Fiona not to jump to conclusions until there was a biopsy result.

During this period she was given so much information that she recalls thinking, 'You realise how little you know and I was listening carefully and I understood only 50% of what the specialist was saying to me.' Fiona understands it is difficult to know when is the right time to give that information as people vary in their approach to how much they want to know and when. She says, 'It is a bit weird when you think, God, I've got a life-threatening disease and yet feel completely fine.'

Fiona found that some days she did not want to hear anything about it and at other times she was desperate to get information and she noted that this changed as time went by. She found there was very little written about bone cancer or sarcomas because it is such a rare disease and there are also so many different types of bone cancer. She was, however, given an information booklet from the hospital and felt that it was helpful. Fiona had many investigations to see if the cancer had spread and a CT scan of her lung showed some suspicious areas. Fiona says this was a difficult and scary time. She said she could cope with having a bone tumour, 'but to think it had spread ... and that I may need chemotherapy.' The specialists – the oncologists and the orthopaedic surgeon – then decided that Fiona should go ahead and have the operation to remove the bone tumour. She underwent a knee and distal femoral replacement, which included a vein graft.

Fiona had expected to be in hospital for about ten days but unfortunately the wound became infected and she remained in hospital for five weeks. After she had recovered, she returned to hospital to have the suspicious areas of tissue removed from her lungs. She was admitted on Thursday and went home on Monday. It was good news: the tissue was not malignant. Fiona feels fortunate that she did not require chemotherapy treatment. After convalescing, she went back to work part time at first and is now back full time and found it was great getting back to normal. She says, 'It's funny how quickly you forget what you have been through. You come to know yourself so well and that is a good thing. I felt I had more inner strength than I probably would have expected. So I now try to enjoy things more, you know. So what if it takes two hours to get to work because there's a tube strike; it doesn't matter in the scheme of things.'

TOM'S STORY

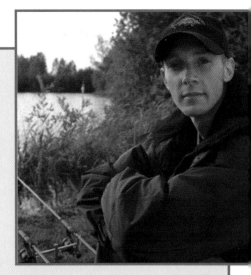

Tom is 21 years old and lives at home with his parents and elder sister. Four years ago, he was fit and active and was enjoying going out occasionally at night with his friends. In the daytime he was working for a bodyshop repairing cars. One day he noticed a lump on his leg. He didn't know how long it had been there but he went to his GP who sent him for a routine blood test and an X-ray at a local hospital. That evening he had a call from the GP asking him to go and see a specialist the following day. 'The specialist said something about sarcomas. I didn't know what that was. I thought I would have a little operation and that would cure it. They were using all these funny names that I didn't really understand. I was only 17 and quite sort of green. My mum, she obviously knew a bit more than I did, but didn't want to let on. It was only when the specialist turned around and said you have a tumour in your leg and it's cancerous - I understood that.'

About a week later Tom was admitted into the Teenage Cancer Trust Unit for chemotherapy. He had a few tests prior to starting the treatment. 'At first I thought the chemo wasn't going to be as bad as they said. Then the next day you think – I don't feel too good today. Then all of a sudden within hours you would be, like, going the other way as well – not too bad. I spent most of my time asleep. I'd come around, have something to eat then I'd go back to sleep.'

Asking Tom how he coped during the chemotherapy he says that the week before going in for the next course of chemotherapy he would try to go fishing with his mates in an attempt to cut off from thinking about the treatment. He found it difficult knowing he would go into hospital feeling well and come out after treatment feeling ill. Because he lost his hair – a side-effect of the chemotherapy – he would cover his bald head with hats. He found people would stare at him and as a result did not want to go out where there were crowds.

Following his chemotherapy treatment, Tom then had an operation on his leg to remove the tumour. 'When I first finished the chemotherapy I said, right, that's it, just check-ups from now on. You think that right now you can start trying to put it behind you and go forward. I had just started to get my life back into some sort of routine when two-and-a-half years later it came back. I was twenty.' When the cancer returned Tom said, 'You feel you are like a piece of elastic in that you get so far away and then you get pulled back.' The cancer had spread to one lung, and was surgically removed.

Tom decided that he didn't want to see a counsellor or the psychologist while he was in hospital having the treatment. He said he felt too ill and had many emotions at that time. He says that while he was in hospital something was being done to help him but that since the treatment had finished it has been the most testing time. He finds that the cancer plays on his mind, he looks down at the scars on his leg in the shower and it is a constant reminder to him. Attending the hospital for check-ups is difficult because, 'You're almost, like, waiting for them to say it has come back again. The anxiety is there under the surface.' Another area Tom finds difficult is not knowing the definite outcome of his illness. 'If you could go into the future and see yourself in ten years, it would be fine.'

For Tom the hardest thing is, 'You just want a cure – but there is no actual cure. I want a definite yes, we've sorted it. But with time you realise that is not going to happen. Coming to the clinic there's no good news, it's only bad news or not so bad news. It's just a case of wait and see.'

These tumours should be treated at supra-regional centres who have expertise in treating this type of cancer. There have been remarkable advances in the management of primary bone tumours over the past 25 years, including the introduction of chemotherapy (now fully established, though new regimens are being tried out all the time) and the development of limb-sparing surgery.

treatment

CHEMOTHERAPY

Most patients should be treated with pre-operative chemotherapy in the first instance, i.e. after surgical biopsy, but before definitive surgical removal of the primary. This not only produces tumour shrinkage (and often tumour cell death) in many patients, but also gives excellent information in each individual case as to the value of chemotherapy and therefore the justification for using yet more, following on after the surgery. For both osteosarcoma and Ewing's tumours, chemotherapy reduces the risk of spread to other parts of the body (this, of course, being the most dangerous and potentially fatal complication).

RADIOTHERAPY

Radiotherapy does not generally play any part in the management of osteosarcoma, but may be useful in Ewing's tumour to mop up what cannot be achieved with chemotherapy and surgery, particularly bearing in mind that Ewing's tumour, one of a group of pathologically similar 'small, blue, round cell tumours' (not perhaps an elegant description, but an accurate one, covering a variety of pathological entities), is an extremely radio-sensitive condition. In some patients with primary Ewing's sarcoma of difficult or central sites such as the pelvic bones, radiotherapy may have to be substituted as the primary form of local treatment instead of surgery, which would be too destructive to contemplate.

SURGERY

For primary bone tumours of the limbs (the most common sites encountered), conservative limb-sparing surgery has dramatically improved the quality of life for these young patients. The whole of the tumour area is removed, taking a fairly generous portion of normal bone as well, and the whole area replaced by a tailor-made, bio-engineered metallic internal prosthesis, allowing complete preservation of the limb rather than, as in the old days, an unavoidable amputation. This is a truly remarkable feat of surgery which, particularly in the case of the lower limb, generally results in an almost normal degree of functional mobility and power. The amount of work that goes into each case is phenomenal, and in younger children with substantial growth potential, a telescopic prosthesis is sometimes used or, alternatively, a planned replacement with a longer one at a later stage. One of the trickiest parts is getting the limb length exactly right, to avoid pelvic tilting and a dissatisfied patient with a lifelong limp. The technique is used both for osteosarcoma and Ewing's tumours, and one or two of the rarer types of bone disorder as well. Most patients require further chemotherapy in the post-operative period.

prognosis

As a result of these new departures, the outlook for patients with osteosarcoma and other primary bone tumours has dramatically improved with at least half of all patients alive and well, probably cured, at five years. Even in patients who do relapse, the use of further chemotherapy (sometimes with very intensive, high-dose regimens and autologous bone marrow transplantation) can be extremely valuable. As previously mentioned, patients with one (or even a few) pulmonary (lung) nodules at a late stage should certainly be considered for surgical removal, since this can still occasionally prove curative.

As the patients are generally young and subject to any number of potential long-term complications, all the points made on page 152 in relation to chemotherapy for lymphomas hold good here. In addition, however, there are other problems. Some patients, notably those with a primary bone tumour situated high in the femur (thigh bone) or parts of the pelvis, will sadly need an amputation of the leg in order to gain control. Obviously this produces special problems of psychological support, follow-up and rehabilitation, too complex to go into in any real depth here. It is remarkable – and uplifting – to see how these young patients cope, and there seems no limit to what they will get up to. We have patients with limb amputation who are proficient skiers, who go rock climbing, sailing and even bungee jumping.

One of the real benefits of a bone tumour centre is the provision of a dedicated teenage cancer ward with all the noisy surroundings and incomprehensible preferences that adolescents seem to need: it really is the case that they are neither adults nor children – particularly not the latter. The expert nursing care, psychological support and medical input as well as activity co-ordinators and teachers on the unit have an important part to play. Treatment should be co-ordinated by those who really are specialists in this work, and there's no doubt that the professional pains and pleasures we experience as oncologists and health care professionals are thrown into particularly sharp relief when dealing with this extremely vulnerable group of patients.

HODGKIN'S DISEASE

causes

Hodgkin's disease is rather a curiosity, since there is no clear agreement as to the origin of the malignant cell. Suffice to say that lymph nodes from Hodgkin's disease usually contain large cells, which are the hallmark of this disorder and thought to be the malignant component – the so-called Reed-Sternberg cell, which has very obvious characteristics under the microscope. The cause is unknown, though there are one or two reports of family clusters, raising the possibility (completely unproven) that there might be some type of genetic or infectious link – of course, it might just be coincidence. The association between Hodgkin's disease and higher socio-economic classes (on standard measures of deprivation) is well documented.

Hodgkin's disease has an unusual age distribution, with one peak around the age of 30 and a second in later life, possibly suggesting different causations for a younger and older age group.

MOST COMMON SYMPTOMS OF HODGKIN'S DISEASE
Night sweats
Fever
Weight loss

symptoms and diagnosis

● The most typical clinical feature is a painless, enlarged lymph node, usually in the neck, but also occurring in the armpit or, less frequently, the groin area.

● Some patients have nodal enlargement in more than one site, and a straightforward X-ray may also show glandular enlargement in the chest even though the patient may be completely unaware of it.

● Often there are no symptoms at all, but some patients complain of night sweats, unexplained fever or weight loss. These are extremely important since they carry prognostic weight, i.e. they affect the outcome and, if present, will almost invariably mean that chemotherapy will have to be used (see below).

● Other interesting symptoms include itching (often widespread) and, curiously enough, pain induced by alcohol often but not always in the site of the lymph node groups involved.

● Although often dramatic, these symptoms are less important than those previously mentioned.

The disease spreads by a fairly logical anatomical progression, generally from the initial area of nodal involvement to the next – neck to chest, for example – but not generally with a skip from, say, the neck to

LYMPHOMAS

Lymphomas are malignant disorders of the lymphatic system of the body, the glands that commonly become enlarged during infections and which are connected by a rich network of lymphatic vessels. To some extent, there is an overlap with certain varieties of leukaemia (the lymphocytic or lymphoblastic varieties), discussed further on page 158. Within the lymphomas, Hodgkin's disease is the most well known (see above) and is so distinct from the other types that the rest are generally referred to collectively as non-Hodgkin's lymphoma (see page 153), though within this latter group there are considerable variations in cell type and clinical behaviour. This group of diseases is, in fact, so diverse that there is a wide division of opinion among pathologists as to how they should be classified; not, perhaps, of overwhelming interest to the non-specialist but of great academic importance, since it is only by classifying tumours in an agreed way that we can possibly compare the treatment results from different centres. Over the past 30 years or so, the outlook for patients with these diseases has improved enormously.

the abdominal lymph nodes. Conversely, patients with groin nodes are unlikely to develop chest disease without abdominal node involvement as well. In more advanced cases, the spleen is involved (about 30% of all patients), sometimes causing splenic enlargement. Involvement of the liver, bone and lung are much less common, around 5% overall.

Staging the disease is extremely important in order to determine the degree of advancement. Stage I denotes a single lymph node site involved; stages 2 and 3 have increasing degrees of involvement (in the case of stage 3, including node groups on both sides of the diaphragm); patients with stage 4 disease have non-glandular involvement (liver, lung, bone, etc.) and are usually suffering from night sweats, weight loss or unexplained fever, often all three. About a quarter of patients with Hodgkin's disease have these symptoms when first diagnosed though not all of these, fortunately, have stage 4 disease.

Very occasionally, the nodes can become so large that they cause pressure symptoms, for instance in the chest, where the patient may have superior vena cava obstruction. Patients with Hodgkin's disease also have reduced immunity, and are more likely than the general population (or other cancer patients) to develop infectious illnesses from viruses, bacteria or even fungal causes.

treatment

The clinical stage of the patient will determine the best form of treatment. All patients should be staged with chest X-ray, blood count and CT scan of the chest and abdomen, to assess the various lymph node groups and also the spleen. Some years ago, there was a vogue for performing exploratory abdominal surgery (staging laparotomy) to check whether the abdomen was involved, but nowadays, radiological staging techniques are relied on.

Patients with stage 1 and 2A disease (A equals no symptoms such as night sweats, etc.) are treated by radiotherapy, whereas patients with more advanced disease require chemotherapy. Occasionally, in patients with stage 2B disease where the symptoms are present but very minor, it might be decided to use radiotherapy alone, particularly in patients where chemotherapy-related side-effects (particularly concerns about fertility) are especially undesirable.

RADIOTHERAPY

With radiotherapy, it is recognised that there could possibly be microscopic spread of disease from one lymph node site to another, so in a patient with, for example, neck nodes on both sides of the neck, all the lymph node groups in the upper half of the body are irradiated with the expectation that this will provide definitive treatment and cure.

Each case must be individually planned, since the lungs must be carefully shielded, being very sensitive to radiotherapy. Particular attention is also paid to the spinal cord (which can also be damaged) and the

ANNA'S STORY

Anna was 27, working in music publishing and with a promising career as a solo violinist. She and her boyfriend lived in a run-down flat and had been talking for years about getting married and starting a family – though never quite getting round to it.

As it was a particularly hot summer, she didn't pay much attention when her night sweats began, nor even when they had persisted for six weeks, to the point where she was forced to change her nightdress at least once, often twice a night. Some of the time, she felt feverish, but this, too, was dismissed. Curiously, she only became really concerned when she'd lost a stone in weight and was so exhausted when she dragged herself into work that the first two hours of each day were a complete wash-out.

Her GP found a gland in the neck and asked (perhaps rather tactlessly), 'How could you have missed a gland the size of a squash ball?' How indeed? All too easy, when viewed in retrospect, to ask these obvious questions. The truth is that we all live with situations that develop gradually – quite apart from the denial we often use as a means of avoiding the unpleasant in so many aspects of our daily lives.

It was Hodgkin's disease, oddly enough a diagnosis that still strikes a note of dread, even though it is among the more curable of tumours. In Anna's case, CT scanning and other tests showed that the disease was confined to the upper half of the body, with abnormally enlarged glands in the other side of the neck as well as the central part of the chest. Her condition was possibly curable with radiotherapy, but it was considered much more appropriate to give chemotherapy, since the typical symptoms (night sweats, fevers, weight loss) implied a more widespread disease.

For the first time in her life, Anna felt totally out of control. She had been an extremely successful music student at Cambridge, had had no trouble passing exams, finding somewhere to live, holding on to her boyfriend or getting her career moving. Suddenly she felt let down, cheated, on the receiving end of – what? All things she discovered she didn't like. She agreed to chemotherapy and, in retrospect, felt that it was the threat of treatment-induced infertility that had most upset her and had clearly focused the severity of the problem in her mind. Mortality she could cope with, but to be rendered infertile, or even the threat of such a prospect, really brought home to her the seriousness of the illness. After just two courses of chemotherapy, her symptoms had completely abated and the glandular lump had all but disappeared. After completing the six prescribed courses of treatment, she then went on to have local radiotherapy to the chest (with a 'mantle' field of radiotherapy) and gradually got herself back to normal.

It is now five years later, with no signs of relapse, and, in all probability, Anna is cured. Although her periods, which had faltered during the chemotherapy, returned to normal, she remained somewhat withdrawn and, unexpectedly, more anxious than ever about her infertility until six months ago, when her periods stopped altogether and, to her amazement, her pregnancy test proved positive.

floor of the mouth, in order to preserve normal oral lubrication. Fortunately, all lymphomas are relatively responsive to radiotherapy, so it is not necessary to go to the high doses required for carcinomas – about two-thirds of the carcinoma dose is generally adequate, with the advantage, of course, that side-effects are fewer, though the wide field of irradiation in a typical treatment for Hodgkin's disease can pose problems. For patients with groin involvement, a similar logic is applied, but to the lower half of the body.

These techniques give excellent results in the majority of patients –

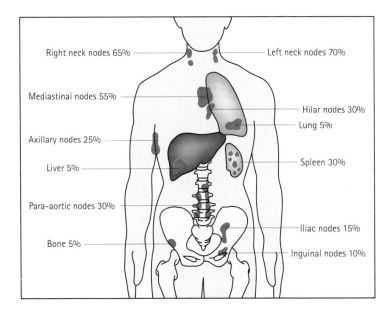

Right neck nodes 65%

Left neck nodes 70%

Mediastinal nodes 55%

Hilar nodes 30%

Lung 5%

Axillary nodes 25%

Liver 5%

Spleen 30%

Para-aortic nodes 30%

Bone 5%

Iliac nodes 15%

Inguinal nodes 10%

Sites of presentation and frequency in Hodgkin's disease. Swelling in the neck and armpit (axilla) are much the most common clinical features.

cure with minimal side-effects. In patients with very localised Hodgkin's disease (stage 1), it may only be necessary to treat the involved area of glands without extending the radiation field; this is perfectly OK provided that the pathology of the tumour isn't one of the more adverse types of Hodgkin's disease (there are several sub-types). The patient should be aware that although cure is likely, there is a risk of involvement of other lymph nodes at a later stage, which will then have to be treated separately, either with more radiotherapy or perhaps with chemotherapy.

CHEMOTHERAPY

All other patients will require treatment with chemotherapy, and this, too, is usually highly successful, with cure as the aim. Hodgkin's disease is extremely responsive to chemotherapy, and the only reason it is not used for all cases is that side-effects, both short and long term, are generally regarded as more severe than with radiation therapy. Fertility, for example, is likely to be impaired as a result of the chemotherapy (particularly in men) and, just as with testicular tumours, patients should always be offered sperm storage if chemotherapy is required.

For young women with Hodgkin's disease, the danger of infertility appears rather less, since the ovaries seem more resistant to the effects of chemotherapy. Many patients continue to menstruate throughout treatment; if so, their chances of future fertility are excellent. In patients who stop menstruating throughout chemotherapy, there is a chance their periods will begin again afterwards (the younger the patient, the more likely this is to happen) and, if long-term infertility should develop, techniques are available at most assisted conception units to help with this. Fortunately, the majority of young women treated with chemotherapy for Hodgkin's disease retain their fertility.

Most treatment programmes involve six or eight courses of intravenous chemotherapy, given every three to four weeks depending on the blood count. Some centres use one programme, some another; many use alternating courses of treatment, i.e. different drugs in the first and second course, and so on, in order to minimise still further the possibility of an emerging drug resistance. There is often an impressive degree of tumour shrinkage, even after the first course or two, and it's certainly possible to cure Hodgkin's disease by chemotherapy alone, though radiotherapy is generally given as well after the chemotherapy has been completed, to the areas of previous bulk disease.

prognosis

Patients with Hodgkin's disease must be carefully followed up since further treatment is usually possible if relapse occurs, and may be curative, even second time round. In patients who are regarded as being at 'high risk', a really high-dose treatment, possibly with the patient's own bone marrow used as support (autologous bone marrow transplantation), is now often considered. This is an exciting area of innovation more fully discussed on pages 57 and 163-4. Patients are sometimes cured by this technique even when all other avenues have failed. Overall, the results of treatment for Hodgkin's disease are extremely good, though patients with adverse features such as anaemia at presentation, high white-cell count or older age, clearly do less well.

NON-HODGKIN'S LYMPHOMA

causes

The non-Hodgkin's lymphomas are a quite different and much more common group of disorders than Hodgkin's disease. The term covers a wide spectrum all characterised by malignant transformation of lymph nodes (but not of the Hodgkin's type or containing the Reed-Sternberg cells referred to on page 148). Within the group, there is tremendous variety both of microscopic appearance (reflecting the varied cell types) and clinical behaviour. Although they are often characterised clinically by lymph node enlargement, just as in Hodgkin's disease, there are many points of difference.
● There is no early peak in age distribution (though there is an important paediatric group of non-Hodgkin's lymphomas).
● A number of congenital disorders are known to predispose to lymphoma in general, of which coeliac disease (a disorder characterised by abnormalities of the lining of the bowel and specific food intolerances) is the most important.
● Non-Hodgkin's lymphoma is also far more common in patients with acquired immune suppression, for example from AIDS or renal transplant anti-rejection medication.
● In some types of rheumatic disorder, notably rheumatoid arthritis and

Sjögren's syndrome (dry mouth and dry eyes from inadequate salivary or tear flow), the incidence of lymphoma is also increased.

● In Africa, Burkitt's lymphoma is a well-known disorder of young adult life which Sir Denis Burkitt (the same surgeon who highlighted the rarity of colon cancer in Africans and linked it to their fibrous diet, see page 110) discovered and described 40 years ago. It is of particular interest to epidemiologists and lymphoma pathologists, since it appears to be caused by an infectious agent (the Epstein-Barr virus), which is likely to be spread by an insect carrier or vector, probably the same species of mosquito that can carry malaria.

symptoms and diagnosis

Non-Hodgkin's lymphoma, or NHL, spreads in a more unpredictable way than Hodgkin's disease. It is far more commonly associated with non-nodal sites, notably the bone marrow, and can also, like acute leukaemia, affect the coverings of the brain (meninges), producing a lymphomatous meningitis.

Although X-ray, blood and scanning tests are important in staging, as for Hodgkin's disease, a bone marrow test will also be required to rule out involvement at this very important site. Although NHL can be classified in a variety of ways – cell of origin, microscopic appearance (morphology), cell size, etc. – pathologists agree that small-cell lymphomas behave fundamentally differently from large-cell ones. Those that form follicular clusters, with the lymph node architecture partly preserved when viewed microscopically, also have a very different pattern of behaviour from the other group, the diffuse lymphomas. Tumour staging systems are similar to those used for Hodgkin's disease (see page 150).

CHEMOTHERAPY

treatment

Truly localised NHL is less common than localised Hodgkin's disease, so the majority of patients with NHL require treatment with chemotherapy. Traditionally, lymphomas with a small-cell follicular-type appearance were regarded as less serious and of lower grade than the large-cell, diffuse variety, since the overall survival following chemotherapy was better. This view has, however, been questioned in recent years because of the effect of chemotherapy, which is different in these two types. In the so-called low-grade tumours, simple treatment, often with tablet chemotherapy, is on the whole as effective as more intensive approaches, though not all lymphoma specialists agree. On the other hand, large-cell diffuse lymphomas respond far better to more intensive chemotherapy, a proportion appearing to be genuinely curable in contrast to the low-grade group in which, at the end of the day, very few if any patients are totally curable, even though lengthy survival is the rule. The question of whether low-grade and high-grade non-Hodgkin's lymphoma should continue to be regarded in the same old way, despite the prospect of curing more patients with high-grade disease, has become a controversial issue.

Detailed choice of chemotherapy depends largely on the cell type.

Low-grade NHL: This generally responds well to simple treatment by mouth and the drug chlorambucil is often chosen. It is usually given intermittently for a week or two, then stopped, then restarted and so on, usually for three to six months, with careful monitoring of the patient's blood count. Sometimes oral steroid therapy is given as well, particularly if the disease proves stubborn and slow in coming under control. For the most part, however, patients with this type of lymphoma, who often have widespread lymph gland enlargement, respond very well. After a few months of treatment it is often possible to discontinue, watch the patient closely and see how things go.

For the most part, low-grade NHL tends to remain fully under control for months or even years, though further courses of treatment are often necessary at a later stage, as they do tend to recur. Fortunately, they often remain responsive to this very simple therapy for years or even decades. Further radiotherapy may be helpful to areas of lymph node involvement and is often highly effective at these sites – particularly useful if there is bulky disease. If resistance to simple treatment does occur later, this can cause real difficulties since the patient will then have to be treated more aggressively, with a less certain outcome, particularly since drug resistance often implies transformation to a more aggressive phase in the illness.

High-grade lymphomas: Here, intravenous combination chemotherapy is essential to bring the disease under control and to offer a prospect of cure. The disease quite often affects young patients (below the age of 50) and, by and large, such treatment is tolerated well, particularly with the advent of powerful new anti-nausea drugs. The precise choice of drugs varies, and because it isn't possible to be absolutely certain of the best choice of agents or intensity of dose, many patients are offered the opportunity of entering a clinical trial in which two or more treatments are compared. With the advent of safer techniques for high-dose therapy, dose intensification is being studied so that the question of whether such treatment gives better results can be definitively answered.

High-dose chemotherapy is more and more widely used in NHL, particularly in patients with recurrent disease who were initially responsive to conventional, multi-agent chemotherapy. Further response to conventional chemotherapy always results in a less durable response than the first time round. With high-dose chemotherapy backed up by peripheral blood stem cell transplantation, the potential range of applications is extremely wide, so in principle, the intensive chemo can be given more than once, for even greater effectiveness. Blood counts will

STAGING NON-HODGKIN'S LYMPHOMA

Stage 1
• Involvement of single lymph node region or single extralymphatic site.

Stage 2
• Involvement of two or more lymph node regions on same side of diaphragm; may include localised extralymphatic involvement on same side of diaphragm.

Stage 3
• Involvement of lymph node regions on both sides of diaphragm; may include spleen or localised extranodal disease.

Stage 4
• Diffuse extra-lymphatic disease, e.g. in liver, bone marrow, lung, skin.

drop quite sharply, generally requiring a three-week stay or thereabouts in hospital before the blood recovers sufficiently for the patient to leave.

RADIOTHERAPY

Since NHL is usually a more generalised type of lymphoma than Hodgkin's disease, radiotherapy has a less important role. Whether or not it is used depends on if there is involvement of the marrow. Patients with NHL often have involvement of the marrow, yet the blood count may be normal. Bone marrow aspiration yields a cellular sample, which can be smeared on to a microscope slide, stained and read very quickly; even more information is provided by a bone marrow biopsy, in which a core of bone is obtained, fixed and prepared in the pathology department. Obtaining a bone marrow aspirate and biopsy is simple.

IVAN'S STORY

Ivan, who is 58 years old, originally hailed from South Africa. He came to the United Kingdom with his wife Esther and two children, a son and daughter, in 1981. He has lived in Britain for 20 years.

In December 1999 he was diagnosed with low-grade follicular lymphoma and his wife Esther had already been suffering from B-cell lymphoma since 1996. She had undergone extensive chemotherapy as well as a stem cell transplant after which she went into remission but unfortunately relapsed after 18 months. At the time Ivan was diagnosed as having lymphoma the family was waiting to see if his wife would be able to undergo a bone marrow transplant. So when Ivan was diagnosed he already had knowledge of the condition and treatments available and was positive he would be cured and was not fearful of the treatment. He began chemotherapy, had three courses and a CT scan which showed no sign of lymphoma. Ivan then underwent two further courses of chemotherapy. After this a bone marrow biopsy was performed and the biopsy sample was clear of the disease.

Unfortunately, in the previous June his wife had become very unwell with relapsed disease. She went on a bone marrow transplant, which was successful but she died from a subsequent lung infection.

During the chemotherapy treatment period Ivan had a blood test, which showed the PSA (Prostatic Specific Antigen) level to be raised (see page 120). The PSA had been monitored throughout treatment but a biopsy on the prostate could not be performed because of the risk of infection and bleeding that Ivan was susceptible to while he was receiving chemotherapy. After the treatment was completed the PSA level was still high and Ivan was recommended to have a biopsy of the prostate. The results revealed prostate cancer and he underwent a radical prostatectomy, which involved the removal of the prostate gland.

Ivan said he had more concerns about the prostate cancer than the lymphoma. He was now a widower and it was daunting to face this new trauma on his own. After the prostatectomy, the PSA level reduced and at the moment Ivan doesn't require any further treatment. He may require radiotherapy in the future and the PSA level will be tested every three months. Ivan also has to have a three-monthly bone marrow biopsy and CT scan to monitor the lymphoma and he has to go through the ordeal of waiting for the results.

Asking Ivan about information he gained or was given on the disease and treatment he says he initially undertook research to understand the treatments that were available to treat prostate cancer but he quickly concluded that the only solution for him was a radical prostatectomy. He says, 'By making sure I understood the nature of the treatment and what the side-effects would be, it gave me a sense of not being

The chosen site is usually in the posterior part of the bony pelvis, the area infiltrated with local anaesthetic, and the needle is pushed in quite firmly and, generally speaking, that's that. The whole procedure shouldn't take more than a quarter of an hour or so, and, in some ways, it's easier than having blood taken, since there's no need to search around for an elusive vein.

If all the tests are clear and the patient really does have a localised form of NHL, radiotherapy is often the treatment of choice; as with Hodgkin's disease, the dose doesn't need to be all that high (see pages 150-2). Treatment does rather depend, however, on the precise nature of the disorder. A high-grade large-cell lymphoma in a young person usually needs treatment with chemotherapy, even if apparently localised, since truly localised disease is unusual. All tests have their

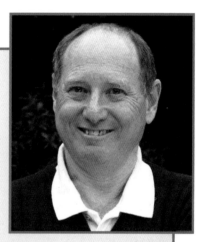

entirely in the hands of the doctors. I had a sense of control over my destiny and therefore focused on getting better, and being positive, thus being able to assist the doctors and the nursing staff as best I could.'

Ivan feels he has recovered very well from the surgery. The side-effects of the operation have been some incontinence and impotence. But the incontinence has improved and pelvic floor exercises have helped this. This impotence is still a problem but because some of the nerves were not damaged during surgery potency may gradually return to normal.

When asked what helped him during this difficult time, Ivan says his wife was helped during her illness with sessions of hypnotherapy so while he was having chemotherapy he and his wife would use hypnotherapy and visualisation together. He has subsequently had two sessions of hypnotherapy, which he believes has been of great help. He tried to remain positive – and visualised the lymphocytes attacking the cancer cells and getting rid of them so he felt he was doing something to help himself. He also feels his philosophy of life has helped. He is Jewish and although he says he is not a religious or observant person in the strictly orthodox sense, he is traditional. He says the interpretation of the story of Job has had an influence on his feelings about what had happened to him and his family and has reaffirmed a philosophy he already had but found he could not articulate clearly.

'People say it's unfair. Why should your wife have cancer and die, and you have two cancers?' Ivan does not see it as unfair. He does not blame God for what has happened. He believes it is nature that has brought about these diseases in his family and he concentrates on the positive rather than dwelling on any reasons for why it happened. Ivan feels that people who find themselves in a similar situation should try to be realistic and understand that cancer can be a fatal illness and that not everyone can be cured. But people can help themselves to remain alive and have a good quality of life for longer and if they can remain so for longer, who knows what treatments will come about to help. 'It is very hard. I've been on both sides of the fence as the relative and the patient, but be positive, it makes such a difference.' Ivan feels it is important to be frank about the illness as very often other people just don't know how to react when they know you have got cancer. 'I found it easier to be totally up front. Tell them.'

limitations, and even the most sophisticated scanners can't always pick up small volume disease at a distant site.

NHL is a relatively responsive form of cancer to radiotherapy and chemotherapy; surgery plays no part in their management, apart from the patient having a biopsy at the outset and if the disease returns and there is doubt as to the nature of the relapse. However, Hodgkin's disease and NHL are both potentially curable and are certainly compatible with a lengthy and normal life. Because of this, it is justifiable to push hard with treatment, even after a second or third relapse, though obviously the greater the number of relapses, the less likely a total or permanent cure.

LEUKAEMIA

The word leukaemia (literally 'white blood') strikes, if anything, an even more fearsome note than the word 'cancer' – understandable, perhaps, since traditionally leukaemia was regarded as both incurable and chiefly a disease that affected children. But the situation has altered drastically over the past 30 years as a result of the development of powerful anti-leukaemic drugs, together with their very careful assessment. Controlled clinical trials from national and international leukaemia groups have led the way in the application of medical and statistical techniques essential for demonstrating that new treatments really are better than what went before.

Although leukaemia is often thought of as being synonymous with an extremely acute, rapidly developing illness in young people, the truth is more complex. Leukaemias are characterised by excess production of white cells in the blood, generally the cells on which we depend for fighting off infection and retaining full immunity; but different types of leukaemia affect different types of white cell (or, more accurately, white cell precursor, since this is essentially a disease of the bone marrow, not only the blood). The characteristics of each type of leukaemia will vary as a result.

the different types of leukaemia

Acute leukaemia is a group of illnesses characterised by sudden and often rapid development whereas the chronic leukaemias are generally much more insidious, slower in onset and not necessarily requiring such urgent treatment. Although red cell leukaemias exist, leukaemia is essentially a disease of excess white cell production and the consequences that follow.

ACUTE LYMPHOCYTIC LEUKAEMIA (ALL)

The most common childhood leukaemia is termed acute lymphoblastic leukaemia (ALL). This term implies a disease of the lymphocytic white cell series, which is closely related to the abnormal cell in non-

---

WHAT IS BONE MARROW?

Since the marrow is the manufacturing site for cells that will circulate within the peripheral blood, there is a whole host of differing red cell, white cell and platelet precursors. Although bone marrow is not evenly distributed throughout every bone in our bodies, it is widely present and mostly exists in liquid or semi-liquid form, which means that not only can a bone marrow sample be taken with relative ease (see page 163), but also that marrow can be collected for therapeutic purposes by multiple punctures (under general anaesthetic) into marrow-rich areas, aspirating substantial amounts of liquid marrow, usually to a volume of about a litre. Bone marrow can be collected in this way for use in transplantation, either to another person, or, after processing, preservation at low temperature and storage (for months or even years), for re-infusion back into the original individual as an autologous marrow graft procedure.

Hodgkin's lymphoma (see pages 153-8). The leukaemic process, however, results in the development of a far more primitive cell (the so-called lymphoblasts – or 'blasts', for short), easily identifiable within the marrow. These essentially represent a highly abnormal, immature and malignant variant of what should have later developed as a normal lymphocyte, and are usually easy to detect. They can be present in such large numbers that the total white cell count on an automated counting machine may be five times greater, or more, than normal.

CHRONIC LYMPHOCYTIC LEUKAEMIA (CLL)

By contrast, in chronic lymphocytic leukaemia (CLL), although the total white cell count may be grossly elevated, the malignant cell type and its degree of maturation and microscopic appearance are all far more normal than in the lymphoblastic variety – so normal, in fact, that patients often feel completely well with this form of leukaemia, often for several years.

Not infrequently, CLL has no symptoms, being discovered by chance when a blood count is taken for other reasons. CLL is closely related to well-differentiated lymphoma and they are often treated similarly – indeed, neither condition necessarily needs treatment at all. This may sound odd, but CLL is often a very stable condition, characterised only by obvious abnormalities in the bone marrow and blood picture, but with normal or near normal immunity and adequate levels of the circulating blood cells, which we all need. About a quarter of all patients have no symptoms at the time of diagnosis, even including some in whom the white cell count is really high, perhaps ten times normal.

ACUTE MYELOBLASTIC LEUKAEMIA (AML) & CHRONIC MYELOID LEUKAEMIA (CML)

The other two major types of leukaemia involve a quite different white cell abnormality. Acute myeloblastic leukaemia (AML) and chronic myeloid leukaemia (CML) involve cells from the 'myeloid' series.

Although these, too, are diseases of the white cell line in the marrow, the maturation and origin of the myeloid white cells are quite different from the lymphoid precursors.

Myeloid stem (or true precursor) cells produce the specific white cells, termed granulocytes, so named because they contain visible granules when stained appropriately and viewed under the microscope. More importantly, they have a specific function in the body, dealing with bacterial infections – pneumonia, bacterial meningitis, soft tissue and wound infections and so on.

Patients with AML and CML are subject to serious bacterial infections because they lack properly mature granulocytes with normal physiology, i.e. the ability to work in the required and proper manner. Their immunity to these infectious diseases is grossly inadequate, and equally seriously, abnormal myeloid precursors often crowd out the marrow to such a degree that, in both AML and CML, the other precursors, producing red cells and platelets (the tiny particles that help the blood to clot), are greatly reduced in number. This produces anaemia and/or thrombocytopenia (i.e. deficiency in circulating platelets).

The same is also true of ALL but rarely of CLL, though this can transform in its later stages to a far more acute and threatening disease. Unlike CLL, CML is an extremely serious condition, and the term 'chronic' is something of a misnomer, since it implies a slowly evolving illness, which can be dealt with using a rather 'laid-back' form of therapy. In truth, however, it is a far more aggressive and frequently fatal illness than its lymphocytic counterpart, CLL.

Most unusually, CML is characterised by a particular and easily visible cellular chromosome abnormality, virtually all cases of CML possessing the so-called Philadelphia chromosome, which is, in fact, a fragment of chromosome 22, first described in 1960. In almost all (about 80%) patients who have been successfully treated for chronic myeloid leukaemia, often by bone marrow transplantation from a sibling donor, this chromosome fragment totally disappears.

symptoms and diagnosis

The symptoms of leukaemia vary with the type of disease. In childhood, ALL accounts for over three-quarters of the cases, with a slight male predominance.

ACUTE LYMPHOCYTIC LEUKAEMIA (ALL)

In childhood, ALL accounts for just over 25% of all childhood cancer in Britain. It isn't exclusively a disease of childhood, however, and is in fact numerically more common in adult life.

● Previous radiation exposure can cause it, a link recognised after the Japanese bomb blasts in 1945.

● It is also more common in children with Down's syndrome, a genetic disorder with an extra chromosome, number 21.

- Symptoms occur as a result of bone marrow infiltration by diseased and functionally useless cells, and include anaemia, thrombocytopenia and infection.
- The history is often brief – only a few weeks of general ill health or malaise, occasionally with fever, sometimes with bone pain.
- With children who have severe thrombocytopenia, blotches, bruises and small red blood spots (purpura) may be visible on the skin; bleeding from the mouth, nose or other sites may occur. Trivial knocks may cause considerable bruising.
- A simple blood count is all that is required in most cases to make the diagnosis (later, of course, confirmed by a bone marrow test).

MOST COMMON SYMPTOMS OF LEUKAEMIA
Fever
Bone pain
Bruising
Anaemia
Fatigue
Irritability
Pallor

CHRONIC LYMPHOCYTIC LEUKAEMIA (CLL)

With CLL, the patient may have no symptoms at all, but the disease is sometimes accompanied by glandular enlargement at one or several sites, or sometimes by recurrent infections, reflecting the reduced level of truly competent circulating white cells.

- The spleen, as well as the lymph nodes, may also be enlarged.
- Non-specific features, of malaise or fatigue, may well be all that the patient complains of.

As CLL is very unusual below the age of 40, it can usually be dismissed as a diagnostic possibility in young people.

ACUTE MYELOBLASTIC LEUKAEMIA (AML) & CHRONIC MYELOID LEUKAEMIA (CML)

The symptoms are often rather similar to ALL, though there are slight differences.

- Most patients with CML have enlargement of the spleen.
- Weight loss and malaise are extremely common, as well as a degree of diffuse bone tenderness.
- Most patients are anaemic and they often, paradoxically, have a rather elevated platelet count, suggesting that whatever is driving the abnormal white cells series may be doing the same thing to the platelet precursors as well.
- In other patients with CML, the platelet count is low, from crowding out of the marrow space by the abnormal proliferating myeloid precursors.

CML typically evolves over a period of months or years from its initial chronic phase to a more rapid transformed phase, in which it is much more difficult to retain control with simple chemotherapy.

treatment

Treatment of leukaemia is different for each of the four main types. In all types of acute leukaemia and CML, the immediate aim is to bring the disease under control with chemotherapy, to reduce the abnormal circulating white count, and, if possible, to obliterate the malignant cell clone within the marrow by chemotherapy.

ACUTE LYMPHOBLASTIC LEUKAEMIA (ALL)

For ALL, the choice and intensity of the drugs doesn't generally have to be quite as powerful or severe in its effect on the patient as is the case for AML. ALL usually responds quickly, often to drugs that aren't too bad from the point of view of serious damage (ablation) to the marrow. Steroid therapy is also used since cells of the lymphocytic series are often extremely sensitive to this very safe agent. It is often possible to produce a virtually normal blood and bone marrow picture within one or two courses of chemotherapy, particularly in a child with the common type of ALL.

CHRONIC LYMPHOCYTIC LEUKAEMIA (CLL)

With CLL, as previously mentioned, there may be no urgency for treatment at all; if there is, it's generally along the lines of therapy as used for well-differentiated or low-grade NHL (see page 154).

ACUTE MYELOBLASTIC LEUKAEMIA (AML)

With AML more intensive chemotherapy has to be given, deliberately ablating the whole of the bone marrow, including the normal elements, with the hope and intention that the normal marrow will regenerate without the malignant clone reappearing. It may take several more courses of chemotherapy to produce the desired result in AML, with a correspondingly greater danger to the patient from each period of bone marrow suppression.

CHRONIC MYELOID LEUKAEMIA (CML)

Traditionally, for CML, relatively gentle treatment using oral chemotherapy was often employed in the first instance, if the patient is in a true chronic phase without evidence of early acceleration or transformation. The appropriate word is 'was' because of the advent of α-interferon, which is now widely used as a first-line therapy; and even more recently, the demonstration of a new and highly effective novel agent, STI-571. This is an incredibly exciting advance in the management of CML – an inhibitor of an enzyme known as tyrosine kinase, given orally as a simple tablet and known by the trade name Glivec. Results have been astonishing, with 53 out of 54 reported patients having a complete haematological response, usually within two weeks of starting treatment, and durably maintained in 51 of these patients. Even more exciting, in a sense, is the emerging principle that this treatment represents, namely the development of a new class of anticancer drugs based on the specific molecular abnormality present in a human cancer.

Since CML may well develop in patients in an older age group, the real difficulty is deciding just how intensive the treatment should be, since it can't be cured other than by marrow transplantation, generally from a sibling donor (or possibly by STI-571, as described above). Treatment of transformed CML by conventional combination chemotherapy (as for AML) sometimes produces remissions, but these are not always long lasting, and a patient with transformed or accelerated CML sadly has a poor prognosis.

Bone marrow transplantation: The good news in CML is that bone marrow transplantation has, for the first time, resulted in true complete remissions and long-term cures, as evidenced by the permanent disappearance in some transplanted patients of the Philadelphia chromosome. This approach has rapidly become the treatment of choice under the age of about 50, if a matched sibling donor is available – though treatment with oral STI-571 may alter this profoundly.

As previously outlined on page 57, in allogeneic transplants, patients are treated with very high (ablative) doses of chemotherapy, and bone marrow from a matched related (sibling) donor is infused shortly afterwards. The object is to destroy the whole of the malignant clone and replace it with 'foreign' bone marrow that is genetically close enough to the patient's own cells not to be rejected. These patients then live the rest of their lives with their brother's or sister's bone marrow in place, a remarkable example of biological hybridisation, since the rest of the body's cells are, of course, the patient's own. Although this is also the case with solid organ transplants, such as heart and kidney, there is no other type of transplant, perhaps, that affects the whole of the body in quite the way that a marrow transplant does.

The technique is also used (in selected cases) in patients with AML or ALL who have relapsed or are at high risk of relapse. Older children or young adults with ALL (particularly males, who do slightly worse than females) who present with a very high white cell count and/or very low platelet count, are of higher risk with conventional treatment, and suitable for bone marrow transplantation during first remission, to try to avoid a relapse ever occurring. In AML, a disease with a worse outlook anyway, bone marrow transplantation (from a sibling or panel donor) is seriously worth considering wherever a matched donor is available.

The difficulties and attendant dangers of allogeneic bone marrow transplantation (even from a closely matched donor or sibling) are much greater than with autologous transplants (see also page 57). Despite the close tissue match, this is after all foreign tissue (unless a genetically identical twin donor is used) and the graft would therefore be rejected unless suitable precautions are taken to induce a degree of tolerance by deliberately producing immune suppression of the recipient (i.e. the patient), using drugs that diminish the normal rejection mechanisms. The problem, however, is that the graft remains immunologically fully competent, and this could lead to a condition known as 'graft versus host disease' (GVHD), in which the graft actually attacks the patient, causing all sorts of complex problems in the liver, skin, marrow and elsewhere. The sophisticated art of successful bone marrow grafting depends on the haematologist maintaining very tight control, with eternal vigilance in the post-transplant period and careful use of the appropriate drugs to avoid on the one hand GVHD, and on the other, rejection of the graft because of an over-powerful level of residual immune competence by the host cells.

The first six weeks or so are quite often stormy, as a result of prolonged myeloid suppression (reduction in the bone marrow capability and cell number) following the very high-dose ablative chemotherapy. Patients will obviously be hospitalised and will usually need intravenous antibiotics, blood and platelet transfusions and immune-suppressing drugs. The object, though, is cure; there is no serious alternative to this intensive form of treatment.

prognosis

For children with ALL, the outlook has improved dramatically since the first effective anti-leukaemia drug (methotrexate) was introduced around 1950. Over two-thirds of children are now curable, but in addition to the initial chemotherapy, they require 'consolidation' and 'maintenance' chemo in order to make sure that the leukaemic clone has truly been abolished. They may also need a course of whole brain irradiation in order to deal with leukaemia potentially developing in the coverings (meninges) of the brain, which isn't adequately protected by standard chemotherapy, hence the need for the radiation therapy. Development of meningeal leukaemia is extremely difficult to eradicate and may well prove fatal in the long run, so it is far better to avoid it.

Testicular irradiation is sometimes used as well (with boys at very high risk because of high white count, etc.) for similar reasons, namely that the testes can act as a 'sanctuary site', which seems to be poorly protected by the circulating leukaemia drugs.

There has been much concern about the psychological, intellectual and physical development of children who have been treated for leukaemia. For the most part they do pretty well. There may be a possibility of a small reduction in intellect as a result, presumably, of the whole brain irradiation, though this is generally minor if present at all. Only very rarely, in an otherwise fit and cured child, does it cut deeply into their quality of life.

The outlook for AML still isn't as good as for ALL, but many patients are cured either by conventional chemotherapy or high-dose treatment with bone marrow transplantation. For patients with AML, irradiation of the brain is not necessary since the disease does not seem to have the same predilection for meningeal involvement.

With marrow transplantation, there is no doubt that the closer the match, the better the results, but even with unrelated donors the level of engraftment is over 90 per cent. Now that the available technology is available, the indications and applications for this type of treatment will increase, as the number of panel donors with known tissue characteristics enlarges. It is worth stressing that the results of matched related (sibling) donor transplantation are better than with unrelated donors, but the probability of having such a donor is, of course, rather low – about 25% – good news for those with large families, but pointing to the need for more research to refine still further the techniques, safety measures and donor panels for unrelated donor transplantations.

MULTIPLE MYELOMA

Myeloma is also fundamentally a malignant disease of bone marrow but it is not, strictly speaking, a leukaemia. In the leukaemias, the whole of the bone marrow is affected, and therefore a sample of any part of the marrow is representative of any other part. In myeloma (or, to be pedantic, 'multiple' myeloma), the abnormal areas develop as abnormal clusters cell within the marrow, hence the use of the word 'multiple'. So in this disease, bone marrow sampling (see page 159), while often important as a means of assessment, is not necessarily reliable since differing sites in the marrow may have a differing degree of infiltration.

Although patients with myeloma have multiple areas of abnormal cell clusters within the marrow, other parts of the marrow are apparently normal. The malignant cell again comes from the white cell series, but is an unusual, large, often pear-shaped cell, quite easy to detect under the microscope. As well as proliferating in the marrow these are capable of directly eroding bone as they grow in their enlarging clumps, causing severe bone loss at specific sites – easily visible on X-rays. As a result, bone pain in myeloma can be extremely severe and widespread, and fractures are common. The disease mostly affects the older age group, usually above 45 years of age. Its cause is unknown.

symptoms and diagnosis

- As with acute leukaemia, both anaemia and reduced circulation of platelets are common, because of the crowding out of the marrow by the malignant elements.
- The most common symptoms of all are anaemia and bone pain.
- There are also all the consequences of a low platelet count – essentially bleeding and bruising – discussed more fully on pages 160-1.

As if this were not enough, myeloma is a particularly unpleasant illness in other ways as well. The malignant cells manufacture and spill into the bloodstream a protein product known as an immunoglobulin, which is normally present in the blood, but in the case of myeloma, at a very much higher level. The type of immunoglobulin reflects the type of myeloma – there are several types, some of which leak the protein predominantly into the urine rather than the blood. The level of this marker can be used to follow progress following treatment – which, of course, can be extremely helpful – but the major drawback is that the protein passes like other blood products through the kidneys. This can severely clog them up, causing kidney (renal) failure and producing

MOST COMMON SYMPTOMS OF MYELOMA

Anaemia
Bone pain
Bruising
Recurrent infections

profound protein loss within the body, since several grams of protein can be excreted in the urine each day as the kidney tubules gradually lose their normal function. Patients who develop renal failure early have a poor outlook; the first and most urgent step is often to reverse this process, if at all possible.

Myeloma patients may also develop evidence of recurrent infections, some of which can be severe and even life threatening. This results both from the reduction in circulating white cells and the fact that the normal levels of circulating immunoglobulins are reduced – despite the single spike of a specific myeloma-related increase in the level of the one characteristic variety. Typically, the other major types of circulating immunoglobulin are reduced, leading to a paralysis of the immune system. This makes it much more difficult for patients to shrug off infections, so they frequently develop urinary, chest and soft tissue infections as a result of the disease process and blood abnormalities.

treatment

Like most malignant haematological disorders of the white cell series, myeloma initially responds very well both to chemotherapy and radiotherapy. Treatment always involves chemotherapy, though there is dispute as to just how intensive the chemotherapy needs to be when first given. The traditional approach is to use melphalan, a simple agent taken by mouth, together with prednisone (a form of steroid therapy), to which the disease is fairly responsive in about three-quarters of all patients. Over the past few years, more intensive chemotherapy regimens have been recommended, particularly for younger patients, and intravenous chemotherapy now tends to be used either together with, or instead of, the oral medication since the initial rate and duration of response are rather better. Apart from chemotherapy, some patients with severe bone pain or fracture will require radiotherapy early on in their illness, together with (or shortly after) the chemotherapy. Orthopaedic pinning is also sometimes necessary.

DEALING WITH REMISSION

Sadly, however, patients with myeloma are generally regarded as having a disease that cannot fully be cured since the disease does eventually return, even if the initial response to chemotherapy was excellent, with significant improvement both of symptoms and substantial reduction (sometimes even to normal) of the myeloma-related immunoglobulin. It might be thought that persisting with more chemotherapy after the initial response should improve the outlook, but in fact there is no point in continuing with more and more chemotherapy when a 'plateau' has been reached, i.e. a situation in which the patient will have improved clinically, with an immunoglobulin level often substantially reduced (though not necessarily to normal).

It is usually best to stop treatment at this point, and to keep a close

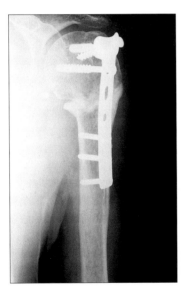

Myeloma deposits are often large enough to cause significant bone erosion. In this patient, the humerus (upper arm) was grossly affected, resulting in a pathological fracture. Treatment was by orthopaedic surgical fixation and post-operative radiotherapy.

eye on things. The conventional approach would be to see how long the remission lasts (typically it is between six months and two years) and then restart treatment when the patient shows evidence of relapse. The use of interferon (see page 213) possibly increases the length of the initial remission, but the point remains disputed. This generally involves three injections a week, usually self-administered, given indefinitely until relapse.

DEALING WITH RELAPSES

When patients relapse, they may well respond again to the initial chemotherapy, but the usual approach is to switch to more intensive chemotherapy. It can be a very fine decision, though, since many patients are well into their seventies, and it becomes increasingly difficult to justify intensive treatment with all the potential dangers. It may be better in some cases to treat the patient palliatively, which generally means local radiotherapy to painful areas (usually extremely successful) and active supportive care, treatment of infection and so on.

Interestingly, the drug thalidomide, outlawed after the recognition that it caused serious birth defects, seems to have a useful role in relapsed myeloma, and is now increasingly used. One advantage is that it can be taken by mouth.

Peripheral blood stem cell transplantation is, however, increasingly given as a means of supporting high-dose chemotherapy (generally with melphalan, this time given intravenously), sometimes together with total body irradiation. This technique (see page 57) has dramatically expanded the potential of this high-dose secondary therapy for relapsed myeloma, since it is simpler than bone marrow transplantation,

HARRY'S STORY

Fitting some high bookshelves one day, Harry, aged 49, stumbled, fell and broke his arm. An X-ray showed that this was a fracture caused within a cancerous area, with clear radiological evidence of thinned and weakened bone. 'Yes, I have had some back pain,' said Harry. 'Quite severe, actually, going back about three months now.' He looked pale, his haemoglobin was about 70% of what it should have been, and a series of X-rays of other parts of the body showed several areas where the bone was eroded. This looked very much like a case of multiple myeloma, confirmed by scrapings from the fracture site, taken at the time of surgical fixation of his arm, and also by the positive bone marrow test.

He was fairly young, and the haematologist felt that he should have intensive chemotherapy with an indwelling intravenous line and intensive treatment, with a view to considering him for a bone marrow transplant if he did well enough. Six months after starting treatment Harry was pretty much back to normal so he agreed to have a bone marrow transplant and three years on Harry is doing well. The prognosis is still uncertain, but so far it looks as though it's all been worth it. For Harry, the only reminders of his illness are the three-monthly visits to the clinic, the regular, thrice-weekly interferon injections he takes and the stiff shoulder.

requires no anaesthetic, and seems extremely safe. Theoretically, there is less risk of contamination of malignant myeloma cells, and there is no risk of GVHD or graft rejection (see page 163) if the patient's own marrow is used. Relapsed myeloma patients up to the age of 65 years or so, for whom conventional chemotherapy no longer has anything to offer, can be treated this way if they are sufficiently fit. The early results are encouraging, and increasing numbers of patients are offered this form of treatment while in their first remission – and without waiting for relapse to occur.

prognosis

With the advent of systemic irradiation, new chemotherapy drugs, interferon, autologous marrow and peripheral blood stem cell support, myeloma is among the most exciting areas of haematology work at the moment. It is an illness where details of management really do matter, and a patient's needs are best served when looked after by an experienced team who thoroughly understand the complications of the disease and are up to date with the latest developments. Myeloma may not be curable, but a great deal can certainly be done to alleviate the patients' misfortunes, often for periods of very many years.

BRAIN TUMOURS

causes

Brain tumours are perhaps the most feared of all human cancers. After all, the brain is the seat of the human mind, widely understood as the most sophisticated of all our organs. How could the body possibly withstand or recover from such a dreadful illness as a malignancy within the very nerve centre of the human frame? They affect both children and adults, varying widely in their type and clinical behaviour. Children's brain tumours are described on pages 182-4.

● For adults, the peak age incidence is 50 to 60 years, and almost nothing is known of the causation or background, apart from the very small group of primary brain, or 'cerebral', lymphomas which can occur in patients with profoundly lowered immunity. For example in AIDS or those in whom long-term suppression of immunity is deliberately produced by medication, for instance in patients with an organ transplant, to avoid rejection of the donated organ.

● These cases are very unusual compared with the far more common group of 'gliomas', a word that embraces the more common types of brain tumour. The term glioma means that the cancer has arisen from the nervous tissue of the brain itself, or the supporting structures within the brain.

● Taken together, these cases account for over 90% of all primary brain tumours (and, for that matter, spinal cord tumours as well, though these are genuinely rare). The characteristic type of tumour in adults is quite different from the childhood types and, overall, a great deal more

---

BRAIN TUMOUR KEY POINTS

Incidence:
About 3,500 cases each year in England and Wales.

Age:
Rare below 30 years but relatively evenly distributed thereafter (peak at age 60 to 69 years).

common. Adult brain tumours rarely spread or disseminate to other parts of the body, a major difference from most other types of cancer. This does not, unfortunately, make them any less malignant, since local control, even by radical surgery and/or radiotherapy, is often extremely difficult to achieve. This is discussed in greater detail below.

symptoms and diagnosis

Symptoms range from the subtle to the devastating – the site of the cancer invariably dictating the pattern of symptoms.

● For example, patients with tumours situated in the highest area, near the vertex of the skull, may have a weakness of the arm or leg, just as if they had had a stroke, since this area of the brain is concerned with motor function.

● Because of 'cross-over' of the major nervous pathways from brain through to the spinal cord, tumours situated in the right half of the brain (the right hemisphere) produce left-sided weakness or sensory loss, and vice versa.

● Even small tumours can produce quite devastating neurological symptoms if situated in the appropriate area, in marked contrast to other sites of the brain where a less critically important area of the brain might be affected. These areas are sometimes referred to as 'silent' areas of the brain, and a good example is the frontal lobe, long known to be the main representational area for personality, intellect and self-control, but with a less clear-cut role in regard to touch, sensation, muscular power or sight.

● Tumours situated at the back of the brain, in the cerebellum or brain stem (situated more or less at the junction of the brain and spine, containing the complicated nervous circuitry passing down from the brain to the varying levels of spinal cord) often produce symptoms of poor balance or more specific syndromes of neurological damage.

● Some types of tumour, notably those in the temporal lobe or underside part of the brain, can cause curious hallucinatory types of epilepsy, in which the patient might, for example, have a very strong sense of a smell which nobody else can detect, a sense of déjà vu, or a foreboding of some terrible impending disaster. One patient with a temporal lobe tumour had overwhelming hallucinations affecting her sense of smell. Unfortunately the smell she experienced was of fire and smoke, and she had raised the alarm and emptied the building where she worked (a large comprehensive school) on five separate occasions before one of the other teachers realised something was up. Patients may liken the olfactory hallucination (i.e. delusional sense of smell) to all sorts of things – strawberries, peppers, acid or, in one odd case (in a wine buff), a 1969 Burgundy. It's all in the brain somewhere!

● Some patients with a brain tumour continually bump into things, from a loss of part of the visual field as a result of the tumour interrupting the visual pathways within the brain. These can be extremely

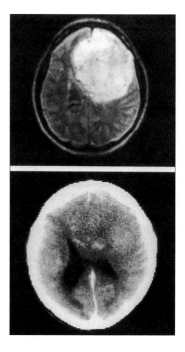

Very large frontal lobe, low-grade brain tumour, which is clearly shown on MRI scanning (top picture) but less distinctly with CT scanning (bottom picture). The initial presenting symptom was a convulsion.

MOST COMMON SYMPTOMS OF BRAIN TUMOURS

Focal neurological deficit 50%+
Seizures 25-30%
Headaches 25-35%
Mental changes 16-20%

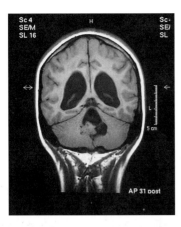

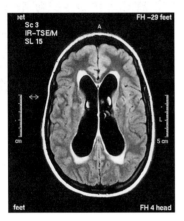

In this patient, the ventricles of the brain, shown as the dark areas deep within the brain substance, are enlarged ('hydrocephalus') due to a small but critically sited tumour, which has obstructed the normal flow of CSF (cerebro-spinal fluid). The top scan shows an image taken across the brain ('coronal plane') whereas the lower one shows the more conventional transverse ('bacon-slice') plane.

dangerous – there are cases where the first symptom was that the patient, normally a careful and courteous driver, repeatedly drove into the kerb or on to the pavement unable to comprehend that a consistent part of his visual field had been lost, so he'd effectively become unable to see out of the corner of his eye.

● The other important groups of brain tumour symptoms are those relating to pressure. It is often not appreciated that the skull is a remarkably rigid structure, which encloses the brain completely. For this reason, any area within the brain that expands – not only from a tumour; it could just as easily be a sudden haemorrhage or clot – will, as a result, produce an increase in the 'intracranial' pressure, since there is simply nowhere for the extra volume to be accommodated. This is the explanation for the frequent complaint of headache.

● Other important pressure-related symptoms include nausea, vomiting and double vision.

● The fluid part of the brain (the ventricles) is in direct communication with the spinal canal and the spinal cord. Any interruption or blockage will lead to increased fluid pressure, and even a small tumour, if situated near the outflow point of the ventricles, is likely to do this, whereas quite large ones located in the outer or more solid part of the brain may not produce these symptoms at all.

● Neurologists and other specialists look for increased intracranial pressure by careful inspection of the back of the eye, since the optic nerve – the nerve from the brain to the retina – transmits the excess pressure with a characteristic appearance ('papilloedema') of the optic disc. Once again, it is the site of the tumour, rather than its precise size or nature, which is likely to determine whether or not these symptoms are present.

DIAGNOSING A BRAIN TUMOUR

The diagnosis of brain tumours has undergone a revolution over the past 20 years, with the advent of CT and then MRI scanning (see page 35). Before these scanners became available, it was necessary to rely entirely on clinical judgement, always a dangerous policy, or to use invasive techniques, which were often painful and could be hazardous. Nowadays, it is possible to gain remarkably detailed pictures with the added advantage that they are safely repeatable after treatment has been completed, to assess what has been achieved.

Apart from the technical quality, the real value of state-of-the-art scanners lies in the enormous advantage they give the brain surgeon or specialist radiotherapist who naturally wish to deal with the tumour as effectively as possible, without disrupting surrounding structures any more than is strictly necessary. Many more tumours can now at least be biopsied more safely than before, giving much needed information on the type of tumour, even though it might still be dangerous or even impossible to go further and remove it entirely. This may involve using a special stereotactic frame, attached to the patient's head, to allow

NON-MALIGNANT BRAIN TUMOURS

Not all brain tumours are malignant. For example, tumours of the pituitary, arising from the hormonally active gland at the bottom of the brain, are always benign. They nonetheless belong to a very important group, since they can produce extremely serious symptoms, either by hormone under- or over-production or by simple expansion leading to dangerous pressure on surrounding structures. Sitting just above and in front of the gland, for example, is one of the most important parts of the nervous network between eye and brain, the optic chiasm. Interruption of this structure can lead to permanent loss of vision, resulting in a characteristic visual field alteration known as a 'hemianopia' because half of the visual field will be lost, and the other half perfectly retained. This is the type of patient, rather like the teacher who had hallucinations affecting her sense of smell (see page 169), who bumps into things or, unaware of the defect, drives into a kerb or lamp-post. Other types of benign brain tumour include those affecting the covering layers of the brain, the meninges; a so-called meningoma is often one of the more gratifying brain tumours to treat, since it is often possible to shell these out successfully by skilled neurosurgery.

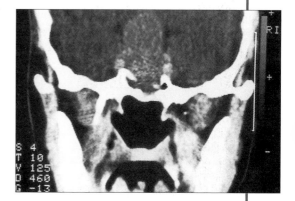

Brain scan showing a large pituitary tumour, seen here as a grey mass growing upwards in the midline from its original site. The base of the skull is also clearly shown. Again, a coronal view.

needle biopsy (under scanning control) of a tumour not amenable to any other type of surgery. This particularly applies to those in the 'dominant' hemisphere of the brain, i.e. the side containing the speech area, generally the left-hand side of the brain. Most surgeons would be much more prepared to remove tumours on the right ('non-dominant') side than the left, though unfortunately brain tumours are as common in the dominant as in the non-dominant hemisphere.

It is generally not too difficult for a pathologist to describe the tumour grade, using a grading system dividing primary brain tumours into four types, from the least to the most malignant. The length of clinical symptoms is likely to be much shorter with tumours of higher grade (3 or 4), but with grade 1 or grade 2 tumours the patient may have suffered a slowly evolving clinical history, often over many years, typically suffering also from epilepsy if the tumour is situated in the appropriate part of the brain. As with so many types of cancer, it is far easier to deal with a small tumour than a large one; indeed, it may even make all the difference between cure and failure. In other cases, particularly for the most malignant types known as 'glioblastoma multiforme', the microscopic appearance, by contrast, shows a much more disordered and bizarre cellular arrangement, quite unlike normal brain tissue, and with a much more elaborate blood supply.

treatment

Although diagnosis of brain tumours has become more straightforward with the wide availability of CT and MRI scanning, the same cannot be said of treatment. There remains a wide variety of views among neurologists, neurosurgeons and oncological specialists, some even taking the view that in high-grade tumours, treatment results are too poor to justify routine intervention, with all the attendant dangers. Others adopt a much more positive approach, following the philosophy that the negative or nihilistic view will inevitably result, sooner or later, in failure to treat a tumour that could have been cured or at least controlled for a lengthy period.

With low-grade tumours, the outlook is not too bad, at least for patients over the age of 50 or so, since many will survive for years or even decades following initial treatment with either surgery or radiotherapy (or sometimes both). On the other hand, those less convinced of the benefits of immediate treatment point to patients with low-grade brain tumours whom they have followed over several years, using repeat CT scanning, but without active intervention unless the tumour enlarges or the symptoms become severe.

Although the matter has never been formally settled by a proper comparative study, it is increasingly accepted that most patients do benefit from early treatment, and there are certainly many cases of low-grade brain tumour in which the patient has struggled for years with recurrent epilepsy symptoms, often very difficult to control, but improved by radiotherapy, even if the tumour was too large or dangerously situated for surgical resection. It is therefore possible to justify treatment on symptomatic grounds, even if an improvement in overall survival cannot be guaranteed.

The same general points apply, perhaps with even greater force, to high-grade brain tumours, where the prognosis is regrettably so much poorer, even with active treatment. Patients with these tumours really do have the cards stacked against them, particularly with the very high grade (glioblastoma multiforme) cases, where cure is very unlikely (though not entirely unknown). But this doesn't necessarily mean that nothing can or should be attempted. First of all, patients with high-grade brain tumours need time, both for themselves and their families, to adjust to a devastating and probably fatal condition; this can only be offered if the specialist can at least recommend or point to a coherent treatment policy. It may be that the patient only has a few months to live, but what important months they are. Secondly, the quality of life is often likely to be improved by treatment.

It is, of course, accepted by specialists that the time spent in hospital following a major brain operation may well interfere with this, and the same applies in principle for radiotherapy attendances. On the other hand, the quality of a life in which the patient knows full well that he or she is simply waiting, often unaided, for the end, seems grossly impaired as well. Active treatment does at least allow for a positive and pugnacious approach which most patients, their partners and families find rewarding at the time, even if ultimately a failure. And then thirdly, you get the odd surprise. For example, a high-flying barrister some years ago, struck down by a very high-grade brain tumour, found it difficult to decide whether or not to agree to active treatment. In the event, he decided to go for it, and lived for another 15 months, much of the time spent on his feet in the courtroom, winning a couple of cases that he had almost given up on, and with the large bald area from the radiotherapy very adequately covered by his barrister's wig. In cases like these, it is often the family who benefit as greatly as the patient. There is nothing so disheartening as feeling guiltily (rightly or wrongly) after the death of a loved one that important approaches might have been left unexplored.

SURGERY

Surgical removal of a brain tumour is sometimes possible, particularly with low-grade tumours arising from the outer parts of the brain, rather than from structures situated more deeply. Surgeons are understandably hesitant about removing large portions of the brain, partcularly in the dominant hemisphere (generally the left side), which is responsible for speech function. Brain tumours in children are often more amenable to surgical treatment, and in any event tend to be lower grade, with a better prognosis than in adults. Most high-grade brain tumours cannot be removed completely, and difficult judgement is required – whether to try to 'debulk' or leave well alone.

RADIOTHERAPY

The drawback for radiotherapy is the inevitable hair loss caused by the X-ray beam passing through the scalp; the higher the dose, the slower the regrowth. Psychologically, however, it is extremely tough for patients simply to accept the prospect of living with the tumour for an indefinite period, and undergoing treatment at a later stage, only when the symptoms become intolerable. The difficulty, of course, is that brain tumours, whether low or high grade, are generally not among the more responsive of tumours to radiotherapy (but with some important exceptions, particularly in the childhood group – see pages 182-5), so the benefits may well be limited.

CHEMOTHERAPY

With regard to chemotherapy, the current view is that while both surgery and radiotherapy are fully established as valuable treatment for brain tumours, chemotherapy has a much more uncertain role. There are no drugs currently available that have a really sustained effect, but those that are available are at least partly effective. The chemotherapy does occasionally cause nausea and vomiting, but the side-effects are in general not too troublesome, and many patients have benefited. New agents are also being tried out in this difficult group of tumours, notably an agent developed in the UK known as temozolamide, a drug which can be given by mouth. More traditional agents are generally used first, and further clinical trials are under way.

DEXAMETHASONE

The other drug very widely used in brain tumours is dexamethasone. This is the most potent steroid available, and, like all of them, is a potentially dangerous agent. However, its results with controlling the symptoms of brain tumours are often remarkable, at least in the short term, and many patients' lives have been transformed. It acts by reducing the local swelling (cerebral oedema), rapidly relieving symptoms of raised intracranial pressure and often improving the patient out of all recognition.

The trouble is that these early benefits of dexamethasone may be short-lived, or blunted by side-effects if the drug is given for too long, since all the disadvantages such as muscle weakness, weight gain, fluid retention, easy bruising and so on come into play. Fortunately, it is usually possible to gradually reduce the steroid dose during the post-operative period or after the course of radiotherapy, so that it can be tailed off completely, generally within six weeks or so after completion of treatment without the terrible symptoms returning. If patients relapse at a later stage, when further radiotherapy or surgery is no longer possible, dexamethasone is likely to be the most valuable drug for palliation of symptoms.

SECONDARY DEPOSITS

The brain is a relatively common site for secondary deposits of cancer. The important difference, of course, is that in these cases, the primary tumour has arisen elsewhere, for example in the breast or lung, and may have spread to various other sites as well. These secondary tumours are quite different in their fundamental characteristics from the primary brain tumours outlined on these pages, and, if biopsied, show just the same characteristics of the original tumour from breast, lung or wherever, rather than the distinctive microscopic appearance of a primary tumour arising from the brain itself. They are often multiple, rather than the typically single abnormality of the primary brain tumour, and are treated rather differently.

Neurosurgical removal: This is rarely worth considering, though there are some important exceptions, notably patients where there is a single secondary deposit, and, best of all, where further investigation shows no other evidence of disease at any additional site, particularly if a lengthy interval has elapsed after the original diagnosis was made. Sadly, this only applies in a very small minority of cases, and for the most part, the treatment decision lies between whole brain irradiation

DOMINIC'S STORY

Dominic, aged 47, is second-in-command of a large public company, divorced and remarried, with two young children. Five years ago, he developed a severe headache, blurred vision and nausea, which, he insisted, were work related. He didn't see his GP until three months later, when pressures of work allowed; the GP immediately sought a neurological opinion from a specialist. A week later, a CT brain scan confirmed a large frontal brain tumour, which was removed by a neurosurgeon and turned out to be a low-grade glioma. He made a remarkable recovery and was back on his feet within weeks.

Four years later, the symptoms returned. Again, he ignored them for six weeks, but his wife insisted that he see the specialist again and was furious to discover that, unbeknown to her, he had discontinued his previous follow-up visits, again due to pressure of work. A new brain scan showed obvious reactivation of the tumour, though the scan from the previous year (at his last follow-up visit) had been normal. This time, the tumour proved unresectable, and a biopsy showed evidence of progression to a higher grade, with a much more serious outlook. The recommended treatment was a combination of radical radiotherapy and chemotherapy, and Dominic willingly participated in a clinical trial of a new form of chemotherapy. Once again, he's back at work, now into his sixth cycle of chemotherapy, given on an outpatient basis. Recent brain scans have shown shrinkage of the tumour following radiotherapy, but Dominic and his wife both realise that the disease could still be partly active, even though he has no symptoms.

Although it's probably the case that not much was lost by Dominic's shoulder-shrugging attitude, doctors are so fond of saying that early diagnosis is the key, that it's difficult to remain reassuring on this point without sounding totally inconsistent.

(usually with dexamethasone support as outlined earlier) or treatment with steroids alone, but without the radiotherapy.

Radiotherapy: This can be very valuable, particularly with tumours that are likely to be responsive, such as secondary deposits from small-cell lung cancer (see page 73). On the other hand, the patient will have to accept some degree of hair loss, though not generally long term since the usual convention, quite properly, is to give only a limited dose so as to avoid treatment complications in what is essentially a palliative (non-curative) situation.

Chemotherapy: Chemotherapy may be worth considering as well.

prognosis

There is no denying that brain tumours do indeed produce devastating symptoms. Hospice and community palliative support teams regard them as being among the most difficult of tumours to deal with, and it's never easy to answer the frequently posed question, 'What's going to happen at the end?' The truth is that many patients drift gradually into an increasingly comatose state, often with little in the way of additional symptoms. A caring general practitioner (if the patient is at home), support from palliative care team or nurse specialists can achieve remarkable quality of symptom control by careful use of dex-amethasone, anticonvulsants and other medications; at the very end, it is sometimes the kindest course of action to withdraw the steroid therapy and permit the increasing pressure within the brain to deepen the patient's coma still further.

As far as cure is concerned, there is no use pretending that brain tumours are truly curable – in the commonly accepted sense of the word – all that often. But there are successes, even with patients with high-grade tumours, of whom a small proportion can undoubtedly be cured, without evidence of further relapse following the initial treat-ment with surgery and radiotherapy. They may constitute only a small minority of the total group, but how terrible to miss the opportunity even with a single case.

Current research efforts are directed towards the increasing use of neurosurgical imaging and resection, the investigation of chemother-apy (including novel agents only just introduced into clinical practice), and the development of new drugs, which might have greater potency. There may be a long way to go, but at least the battle is joined.

CANCER FROM AN UNKNOWN PRIMARY SITE

causes

It sometimes happens that a cancer, which is quite clearly secondary in nature, develops without conclusive evidence as to the primary site. Though this is fairly unusual, there are two well-known clinical syn-dromes. The first includes patients with lymph nodes in the neck (or elsewhere in the body, but the neck is a typical site), which are con-firmed at biopsy as squamous carcinoma; and secondly, the patient with diminished appetite, weight loss and mild jaundice who is revealed, on simple ultrasound scanning, to have multiple secondary deposits in the liver, usually turning out, after a simple transcutaneous needle biopsy (through the skin), to have an adenocarcinoma.

Both of these types of clinical situation occur from time to time in the complete absence of symptoms that might point towards any of the likely primary sites, and in every possible sense they are a real problem. To the patient they are a problem because facing cancer is always hard enough without the added burden of realising right from the outset that cure is extremely unlikely. To the doctor and nursing staff it is hard because a kind-hearted and supportive explanation of the true situation is never easy, particularly since so much weighty information may have to be given at the very first meeting between patient and staff. Furthermore, patients find it particularly difficult and terrifying that such a situation could arise without them detecting any symptoms – sometimes feeling as if, in some way, it was their own fault that they simply failed to notice.

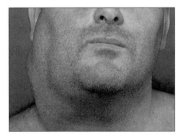

This very large mass in the right side of the neck was obviously a secondary deposit in a group of cervical lymph nodes. The primary site was almost certainly within the head and neck region, probably nasopharynx or oropharynx, but we never knew for sure.

A diagnosis of cancer is hard enough, but when the cancer appears first of all at a secondary site, it seems even more incomprehensible, and is even more difficult than trying to come to terms with a more conventional cancer, which at least had the good manners to declare itself first at its initial point of departure. Unfortunately, the team in charge can't even outline to the patient a plan of management along the usual logical lines – surgical biopsy, staging to check for secondaries, consideration of the best form of local treatment, etc., etc.

It is important, however, at least to make a diagnosis of what pathological type of tumour is being dealt with. A gland in the neck containing squamous carcinoma cells, for example, may well arise from a previously undetected head and neck site, such as the tonsil or floor of mouth, under the tongue – readily apparent on expert examination, which might require an anaesthetic to be completely thorough. If this does confirm a primary site (quite a common clinical scenario) then treatment of the primary site and the neck is well worthwhile, and may even be curative.

An enlarged gland in the armpit (axilla) may well prove to be an adenocarcinoma, and it is extremely important to search carefully for a primary within the breast on the same side, since breast cancers may be very small and undetected by the patient, yet still have the potential to produce malignant involvement in the axillary lymph nodes (this is discussed further on pages 88-9). Even if there's no obvious lump in the breast, it is important to request a mammogram if you are not automatically offered one. This may show the typical features of primary breast cancer, and the management can then proceed in the usual way.

In the case of the liver example given earlier, there is no point pretending that the situation is anything other than extremely serious right from the outset, since liver deposits cannot on the whole be cured. However, there are a few very rare exceptions, since one or two types of malignant tumour can spread to the liver, yet prove later to be strikingly responsive to chemotherapy. So it is always worthwhile trying at least to define the pathological nature of the problem. To achieve this a liver biopsy will need to be performed. This is generally a straightforward affair, and simply involves a needle biopsy carried out under local anaesthetic.

Treatable cancers that may sometimes appear as secondary deposits from an unknown primary site include:

- Breast (see pages 85-103).
- Colorectal (see pages 110-15).
- Ovary (see pages 75-85).
- Prostate (see pages 120-2)
- Small-cell lung cancer (see pages 70-4).

In addition, there are the following three curable tumours that really mustn't be overlooked since they can sometimes be treated very effectively. They are:

- Testicular germ cell tumours (see pages 123-7).
- Thyroid cancer (see pages 139-40).
- Lymphoma (see pages 148-58).

PALLIATIVE TREATMENT

Even where cure is not possible, palliation, either by chemotherapy or (in the case of breast and prostate cancer) by hormone therapy, may be very worthwhile and add substantially to life expectancy. This is particularly important in the case of patients who are likely to survive only a shortish time and may have much to attend to during those few precious months.

In patients who have secondary deposits from an unknown primary site, the whole of the clinical, emotional and evolutionary pattern of cancer is telescoped into a much shorter time than usual, and it is important not to miss these opportunities to try to come to terms with what may well be a short survival time. Perhaps the most important, strictly medical, point is that it is always worth reviewing the pathology very carefully, just in case there is any question of it being a curable or at least potentially treatable tumour. The patient will need a specialist who can offer both experience and support in this most difficult of situations.

Sometimes the patient surprises the team in the best possible way. We have certainly seen patients who, given an almost hopeless diagnosis and a short life expectancy of a few months, have responded to treatment surprisingly well and gone on to live for two or three years. This applies both to patients who have secondary deposits from an unknown primary site and also to the much more common group of patients who develop metastases from a clearly recognised primary site. For example, the patient with secondary deposits in the liver, but no known primary site even after extensive investigations, responded remarkably well to combination chemotherapy. In cancer, the tempo of disease varies in the most remarkable way – so much so that it is usually unwise to be too specific about prognosis, even where metastatic disease has established itself at widely disseminated sites.

SITES OF METASTASES FROM AN UNKNOWN PRIMARY SITE

Site of metastasis	Likely primary site
High cervical nodes	Head and neck sites
	Thyroid
	Lung
Lower cervical nodes	Head and neck
	Lung
	Breast
	Gut
Axillary nodes	Lung
	Breast
Skin	Breast
	Lung
	Melanoma
Bone	Myeloma
	Breast
	Kidney
	Prostate
	Lung
Brain	Lung
	Breast
	Prostate
	Melanoma
Inguinal nodes	Vulva
	Anorectal
	Prostate
	Ovary
Disseminated intra-abdominal adenocarcinoma (including liver metastasis)	Ovary
	Stomach
	Pancreas
	Gut

CANCER IN CHILDREN

There cannot be many more poignant situations in medicine – or life in peace-time – than the diagnosis of cancer in a child. One of every parent's greatest nightmares, it's often viewed as incomprehensible when it actually happens and well nigh impossible, for some parents at least, to take in. Yet the outlook in children's cancers has improved immeasurably over the past 25 years, and as Gary Lineker points out in his Foreword, *seven out of ten children today are completely cured* – perhaps the most important take-away message of this whole chapter, since, tragic though it may be, the diagnosis of malignant disease in a child does generally carry with it at least a genuine and realistic message of hope. In particular, the two most common types of childhood malignancy, leukaemia and brain tumours, are now much more commonly curable than ever before as a result of countless advances, some dramatic, others plodding and painstaking, in all branches of paediatric oncology. As stressed in a handbook for oncological trainees:

'The diagnosis of cancer in a child is an exceptional and painful test to the strength of family life. Happy families often cope better with the shock, grief and disruption . . . Over half of all children with cancer are cured; with many diseases, a cautiously optimistic account can be given. The parents will sometimes feel angry about the diagnosis . . . Often they feel that they have been responsible in some way, in that there is a genetic factor to which they have contributed, or that the cancer has arisen as a result of avoidable physical or mental trauma or faulty diet. They need to express these feelings and must be reassured that they are not to blame.

'Talking to children and their parents requires tact, humanity, patience and a clear head. Every new case will prove an additional test of these qualities, and the doctor and multi-disciplinary team caring for and treating the child will have to deal with the guilt, anguish and anger of the parents, as well as the physical and emotional suffering of the child. All children, except for the very youngest, need some account of why they are in hospital and what is likely to happen, and with older children and adolescents, these explanations will need to be accurate and complete.

'It is impossible to make any generalisation about how much to tell. Children of six to eight years will understand that they are ill and grasp the elements of treatment. At 10 to 11 years, they will know more, and teenagers will know about cancer and leukaemia . . . For children of about 11 years or more, a personal and private relationship with the doctor and nurse specialist is important. They often want to ask questions directly and . . . at times, may feel that the truth is being filtered by their parents. The doctor should try to encourage the family to be open with each other with respect to the illness. Honesty and frankness

CANCER IN CHILDREN KEY POINTS

• Approximately 1,200 children aged under 15 years in England and Wales are diagnosed with cancer each year, giving a rate of 12 per 100,000 children less than 15 years old.

• 1 in 550-600 children will be affected by the age of 15 years, which is similar to the rate for Down's syndrome, diabetes or meningitis in childhood.

are important . . . whereas glossing over of the facts will leave them with insufficient detail to help them understand the implications of the diagnosis and treatment.' We have included this quote, which was part of the general advice given to the profession, in the hope that it is helpful to patients, parents and families. The complexity of treatment of children's tumours makes it difficult to provide detailed answers to all the questions that a parent or child might ask, especially at the first consultation. It is essential that an experienced clinician should be in overall charge, though additional specialist advice may sometimes need to be sought – orthopaedic, neurosurgical and so on. This then permits that most important feature of care, the identification by both patient and parents with a single individual rather than a committee.

JONATHAN'S STORY

Jonathan is a 15-year-old teenager from south-east London who lives at home with his mother, his two brothers (aged 13 and 17 years) and his sister (aged 11).

Jonathan had a lump in his foot, which gradually got bigger. After a few weeks he went to his GP. He was then referred to a specialist and a biopsy was performed to obtain a diagnosis. Jonathan was with his Mum when they were informed that the biopsy result showed that it was a synovial sarcoma. Jonathan recalls, 'It was a complete shock and totally unexpected.'

Jonathan quickly underwent treatment, which consisted of six courses of chemotherapy, one every three weeks, which meant that he usually went to the Teenage Cancer Trust Unit at the hospital on a Friday and returned home after completing treatment the following Monday.

Jonathan says the worst thing was the side-effects of chemotherapy some of which were so unpredictable – he felt absolutely terrible and was 'run down and groggy' most of the time. He was informed that the type of chemotherapy he had meant he would lose all of his hair but that it would grow back after treatment was completed. After the first course of chemotherapy he asked one of his brothers to shave off all his hair for him so that he wouldn't see the clumps of hair falling out. Jonathan found that losing his hair was very difficult. He refused to let anyone see him without it – he wore a woollen hat all the time, even when he slept, and only took it off when he had a bath. Now his hair has re-grown and has come back with a bit of a wave and is softer than before and he says, 'It hasn't changed colour – all those stories I heard "Oh it's going to grow back ginger or blue!"'

Talking about support during his treatment Jonathan found he talked mainly to his Mum. He didn't want his brothers and sister to come and see him in hospital while he was in that condition. Asked why, he said he was embarrassed and also that he was keeping it all from them and possibly protecting them. He felt he did the same with his friends and says, 'It's not their fault they don't know a lot about it – they know it's cancer and they know it's serious but they don't know what it entails.'

Asking him if he talked to the other teenagers on the ward he replies, 'No. I think if you went now and asked the ward staff they would say that I had the curtains pulled around my bed 24 hours a day and that I wanted to stay in bed all day too. I didn't want anyone to see me. I don't know why, I wasn't used to being laid up like that.'

Jonathan says he never really wondered why this had happened to him; he never had self-pity or felt sorry for himself. He has found that his religious belief and faith have helped him. 'It keeps me sane because I

This is not primarily a book about childhood cancer, so it would be unwise to attempt too much detail about the specifics of paediatric malignancies. Although they are all uncommon, cancers are the most common natural cause of death in childhood, after domestic and road accidents, which sadly still come top. As previously mentioned, the most common types are leukaemia (chiefly ALL – see pages 160-1) and brain tumours (see overleaf). Non-Hodgkin's lymphomas (discussed on pages 153-8) are also relatively common, though Hodgkin's disease is very unusual (see pages 148-53). The other types common enough to merit discussion here are neuroblastoma, Wilms' tumour, retinoblastoma, and finally the paediatric sarcomas, which are in some respects slightly different from the adult diseases discussed on pages 142-8.

believe in life after death and I feel this isn't the end anyway. No, I'm not frightened – to tell you the truth I'm more worried about my Mum and family. I'm not worried for myself at all really. I can say that that is the truth. If religion was not part of my life, and it has always been so, then I would have nothing to turn to. When you have an illness like this, it's good to turn to something, which I have done, but not in an obsessive manner. I'm a normal person. I've just got that side to me as well. I'm not ashamed to admit it.'

Asking Jonathan what would have been helpful to him during this time he feels that his friends could have contacted him a bit more and been a little more pushy. When he questioned why they didn't phone him he found it was because they didn't know what to say. Jonathan is now getting together with his friends more and says, 'They can see that I am the same old person.' He felt isolated to some extent during the treatment period and says that 'really you need to be with your own age group.'

Unfortunately, the cancer has spread to Jonathan's lung and he has made his own decision to have 'no further chemotherapy as it won't cure the cancer. I asked the specialist and he said it won't permanently cure it, so after a lot of pros and cons I finally came to the decision and I think it is the best decision really. I'm feeling the best I have felt in months.' Jonathan has, however, consented to having some radiotherapy treatment to try to relieve the pain caused by the tumour in his shoulder.

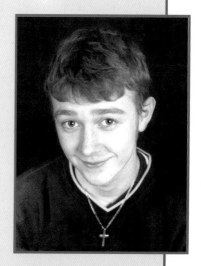

'I know I'm not going to get a miracle cure. I know what is going to happen to me and I am prepared for it. I'm accepting my condition. It was the hardest thing ever to decide whether to have more chemotherapy treatment. I could have gone through more chemotherapy if there was the faintest chance of a cure but there wasn't. There are only two options – the same is going to happen anyway. So that was my decision but a lot of thought went into it.' Looking back, Jonathan says, 'Obviously it is not the nicest of experiences to go through but you cannot choose what is going to happen to you.' When Jonathan is asked what he has planned for the next few months he says, 'I think I will just go on as normal. I don't go to school as they are doing their GCSEs but I go out with my friends. I wouldn't normally go to Disney World so I'm not going to do it now. I'm a realist but I'm not a pessimistic person. I think you should rely on yourself and try to make your own decisions just like I did.'

BRAIN TUMOURS

Paediatric brain tumours differ in several important respects from the adult group, covered on pages 168-76. The most common single type is medulloblastoma, a tumour which is rarely seen over the age of 25 and arises from the back of the brain, the cerebellum, with a peak age of

PAUL'S STORY

Paul was one of those active nine-year-olds who could never sit still. Skateboarding, mountain biking, sponsored swims – he'd embraced them all with equal enthusiasm. But he seemed to be developing an odd kind of clumsiness, a tendency to fall, which eventually became quite exasperating. On the first visit, the doctor couldn't find anything specifically wrong, but a month later, when Paul had had two more falls in the street playing after school, his mother took him back and insisted on a more thorough examination. When the doctor asked Paul to walk heel-to-toe in a straight line, it was immediately clear that the task was quite beyond him, and an urgent referral to the local paediatrician was followed within a day or two by a brain scan.

It was quite a large tumour, bang in the midline, almost 3 centimetres across. Clearly it was a case for the specialist paediatric neurosurgeon; fortunately, he seemed pretty confident that it could be removed without too much trouble.

It turned out to be a medulloblastoma, the most common of the childhood brain tumours arising in that part of the brain. The brain surgeon explained that the tumour had indeed been removed entirely, but that this wasn't in itself sufficient to provide a confident cure and that radiotherapy would be required as well. For his part, the radiotherapist seemed in two minds about whether or not the radiotherapy should be supplemented by chemotherapy, but eventually opted for radiation alone, explaining to Paul's mother that these tumours had a tendency to seed down the spine, and therefore treatment should include not only the brain, but the whole of the spinal cord as well. It all seemed a lot to take in, particularly since Paul's mother was a single parent with two other children (one with Down's syndrome, the other with troublesome intermittent asthma) to take care of. She was particularly concerned about the discussion of possible side-effects such as growth failure and maybe even a fall-off in Paul's school performance – but there didn't really seem to be any choice.

The treatment went well; Paul's uncle was a taxi driver and was able to fetch and carry without too much difficulty. After the surgery, Paul had been extremely floppy and cantankerous for a few weeks but seemed to improve during the radiotherapy, or at least the first part of it. Towards the end, though – it was a taxing, eight-week course of treatment – he was beginning to tire easily and spent most of his afternoons in bed. It took the family quite a while to readjust to completion of treatment and the possibility of a more normal life again. Paul's mother found the first anniversary of his diagnosis absolutely nerve-wracking. But physically he seemed fit enough, and the cancer never reappeared, though it was an anxious time for the whole family, particularly when follow-up visits and scans were due.

Paul is now 14 years old and seems well; the oncologist is almost certain that he's cured. He attends for follow-up at a special growth clinic, since he needed growth hormone injections from shortly after the completion of radiotherapy until a few months ago. His final height looks like being just two inches below the initial predicted figure. Indeed, puberty, too, seems to have been normal and unaffected by the treatment. A year ago, Paul started a Saturday job in a local bike shop and seems as keen as ever on messing about with grease and crankshafts.

about four to ten years and a two-to-one male predominance. It forms about 30% of all brain tumours.

The symptoms result from disturbances of the functioning of this part of the brain.
● Some patients have symptoms of raised pressure as well – headache and vomiting, particularly in the morning.
● The chief function of the cerebellum is to maintain co-ordination and balance, and specific symptoms are therefore likely to include abnormalities of gait – shuffling, falling, difficulties in walking or running, increased clumsiness.

One of the most sensitive tests of cerebellar function is the heel-to-toe walking test (beloved of TV and real-life police officers though they, of course, normally perform the test for a different reason). In a child, persistent headache and vomiting, and inability to perform the heel-to-toe walking test properly should be taken seriously, though there are many causes of cerebellar disturbance other than a brain tumour, including viral infection, etc.

An urgent CT or MRI brain scan is essential and, if abnormal, referral to a specialist is obviously the next step. A brain surgeon (neurosurgeon) will need to be consulted and the child operated on quickly. In some cases, if there is raised pressure from the tumour blocking off circulation of normal brain fluid, a draining shunt will need to be inserted into the fluid space (ventricle) of the brain to reduce the pressure and allow the operation to proceed safely. These tubes can remain in place for many years and rarely give problems. Shunt insertion is often an essential prelude to successful removal of the tumour.

MOST COMMON SYMPTOMS OF BRAIN TUMOURS
Headache 65-70%
Vomiting 65-70%
Changes in personality/mood 45-50%
Squint 20-25%
Behaviour out of character 20-25%
Deterioration in school performance 20-25%
Growth failure 20%

Cerebellar medulloblastoma: Neurosurgeons are almost always able to remove a typical cerebellar medulloblastoma. The child is likely to be in hospital for ten days or so, and in the post-operative period, will need referral to a radiotherapist because surgery alone is never enough. The good news, however, is that the addition of radiotherapy as routine treatment for these children has resulted in a five-year survival rate of about 60%, with most of these children cured and very few relapses beyond this point. Medulloblastoma is probably the most responsive of all brain tumours to radiotherapy, which is used not only to mop up any residual malignant cells that may have been left behind post-operatively, but also to give protective treatment to the spine.

Like a number of other less common childhood brain tumours, this one can seed down into the central spinal fluid (CSF), forming secondary deposits in the spinal cord, though not, as a rule, anywhere beyond. Spinal MRI should always be performed in this disease and all children will need prophylactic radiation therapy to the whole spine, in order to

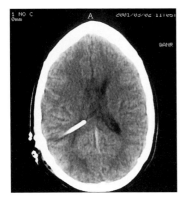

Quite often in a childhood brain tumour, the site of the cancer produces obstruction to the flow of CSF (cerebro-spinal fluid) with subsequent hydrocephalus (see also page 170). Surgical insertion of a shunt, as above, will release the pressure and improve symptoms while the best treatment is being planned.

protect the spinal cord from developing these seedling types of secondary tumour. This may seem like a very tall order, and the treatment does cause problems. For a start, it takes about two months to complete, with the children lying very still. The skill of the radiographers and other staff treating children in special centres is phenomenal – just think about trying to persuade a fretful four-year-old to lie still, preferably without anaesthetic or sedation, for 10 or 15 minutes every day for eight weeks! The radiographers are the real heroes and heroines of the whole endeavour. During this period, the blood count may well fall as a result of the spinal irradiation, and a careful watch must be kept. Total hair loss will always occur, since the whole of the brain will need to be irradiated, though fortunately this is always reversible, and the typical thick hair of a child usually grows back pretty fast.

Some centres recommend chemotherapy as well, generally at a later stage after the radiotherapy is completed, though this form of treatment is not fully established.

Other brain tumours: These do occur in childhood as well, and many require less formidable treatment than the full cranio-spinal irradiation described above. The long-term outlook for children with brain tumours is on the whole considerably better than with adults.

prognosis

In the longer term, children treated by extensive cranio-spinal irradiation are likely to have a number of potential long-term side-effects.

Growth delay: In the first instance, treatment both to the brain and spine are bound to produce a slowing down in normal growth, partly due to the direct radiation effect on the spinal vertebrae within the path of the beam, but also from radiation to the pituitary gland lying at the base of the brain. Growth delay is an almost inevitable consequence of this type of radiotherapy, but can generally be detected quite quickly by means of careful assessment in a growth clinic after treatment – an essential part of the management of any child with medulloblastoma. If growth delay is confirmed, the child can be treated effectively with injected growth hormone, which should restore, almost to normal, the potential loss of height. Growth hormone is now available as a fully biosynthetic substance, so there is no longer any danger of viral transmission, as was previously the case.

Underactive thyroid gland: In addition, the thyroid gland may also become under-active as a result of the X-ray beam passing through the spine out through the front of the neck where the thyroid gland is situated. If this does happen, it is generally easy to correct with thyroxine replacement tablets, fortunately required only in a small minority of patients.

Delay in sexual development: Some children will become slow to develop sexually at the time of puberty, due again either to pituitary failure or, in the case of girls, to a scattered dose of radiation directly to the ovaries, though these are usually situated sufficiently far towards the edge of the pelvis (on both sides) that the relatively narrow spinal beam misses them altogether.

This, too, is generally treatable by the appropriate hormone injections or tablets when the time comes, and fertility is likely to be preserved after cranio-spinal irradiation, even if the child, now of course a young adult, needs help of one kind or another, for example from a hormone specialist. However, these thoughts are usually far from the mind of the parents and child, aged around seven or eight and faced with a potentially fatal brain tumour.

Most of the psychological and developmental studies performed later on, to test whether or not these children are impaired intellectually by the treatment, have been reassuring. If there is an intellectual deficit from treatment to the brain, it seems on the whole relatively minor, though obviously, with more successes there are more children to study and compare with the normal age group. Overall, survivors of this complex form of treatment nearly always grow up to be pretty normal, often with little or no evidence of physical or mental handicap of any kind.

LEUKAEMIA AND LYMPHOMA

The leukaemias and non-Hodgkin's lymphomas of childhood are sufficiently similar to those of adult life not to require much further discussion here. The common childhood leukaemia is acute lymphoblastic leukaemia (ALL), the form of acute leukaemia with the best outlook, and its management is outlined on page 62. In the non-Hodgkin's lymphoma (NHL) group, management again follows the principles outlined for adults (see pages 155-8), but it is worth mentioning that there is even more emphasis on chemotherapy and a move away from radiotherapy in children, to avoid late radiation side-effects wherever possible. Most childhood types of NHL are responsive to chemotherapy.

LEUKAEMIA IN CHILDREN KEY POINTS

Incidence:
245 cases each year in children aged 2 to 4 years in England and Wales. Acute leukaemia accounts for about one-third of all childhood cancers.

NEUROBLASTOMA

Neuroblastoma is the next most common childhood tumour, over three-quarters of cases occurring below the age of four years. This is a curious tumour that arises most frequently from the adrenal gland, the organ situated just above the kidney and responsible for producing cortisone, adrenaline and other hormones. Neuroblastomas are tumours of the particular part of the gland which manufactures adrenaline and similar bio-active compounds, though fortunately, neuroblastomas are not generally associated with high circulating levels of adrenaline.

MOST COMMON SYMPTOMS OF NEUROBLASTOMA

Abdominal mass
Fever
Malaise
Weight loss
Anaemia

symptoms and diagnosis

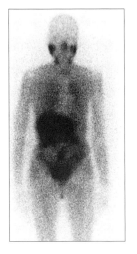

Neuroblastomas sometimes take up a substance known as MIGB (meta-iodo-benzyl guanidine), which can be helpful for staging – using the radioactive version to help locate \ secondary deposits, which might otherwise be undetectable.

- The most common symptom is an abdominal mass (or distension), often surprisingly large, and generally (though not always) painless.
- Affected children are often lethargic and irritable, and sometimes anaemic.
- Neuroblastomas occasionally arise at sites other than the adrenal gland, because of the pre-birth developmental pathway of similar tissue at other sites in the body, so affected children don't always have an abdominal mass.
- Occasionally, lymph node (glandular) or skin deposits are the first clinical sign, or even enlargement of the liver, which is sometimes noted by a parent or the family doctor.
- The tumour can spread widely by local, lymphatic and blood-borne circulation of tumour cells, giving rise to secondary deposits in the liver, bone or marrow, though not generally the lungs.

The diagnosis is confirmed by biopsy (usually of the primary abdominal mass). In addition, because of the embryological derivation of the tumour cells, it is possible to pick up metabolites (break-down products) of the hormones that the adrenal gland produces. Random urine samples – or, better still, a 24-hour collection – are diagnostically helpful. A plain abdominal X-ray is a useful test as well, often demonstrating calcium deposits (calcification) in the primary tumour, and also in liver secondaries, if present. Bone scanning should also be done since the skeleton is such a common site of secondary disease, and a bone marrow test is essential, since about 40% of children with neuroblastoma have marrow involvement even when the bone X-rays are normal.

treatment

Treatment is by surgery and/or radiation, together with chemotherapy in the more advanced cases. Localised cases can often be cured with surgery alone (or with post-operative irradiation, if necessary). If chemotherapy is required, it will sometimes involve intensive treatment with bone marrow or peripheral blood stem cell support, as described on page 57. Unfortunately, neuroblastoma is one of the childhood disorders in which chemotherapy has made only a limited impact; responses are less durable than with some of the other types of paediatric cancer. Its degree of involvement within the body at diagnosis gives an accurate picture as to the likely outcome.

prognosis

Patients with localised disease are usually curable, but if the disease has spread beyond the primary site and its immediate surroundings, this is very difficult to achieve. Newer drugs, more intensive approaches, bone marrow transplantation and so on, may all be suggested, possibly within the context of a controlled clinical trial.

Following successful treatment, most children live a normal life, with far less in the way of potential growth failure and other hormonal abnormalities than is the case for children with medulloblastoma (see page 152). They do, of course need to be followed up carefully, since many of the drugs could have long-term consequences – likewise the radiotherapy, if used, may cause local growth problems at a later stage.

WILMS' TUMOUR

Wilms' tumour (sometimes called nephroblastoma) is a developmental tumour of the kidney, virtually restricted to children, with a peak age of incidence around three to five years and a few cases recorded at birth. Although a little less common than neuroblastoma, it has a better outlook, even though in some cases, virtually the whole of the affected kidney is involved by the tumour process. Pathologically it has an appearance quite distinct from the adult type of kidney (renal) tumour. In about 10% of cases both kidneys are affected and in a very small minority, more than one family member, strengthening the evidence that Wilms' tumour is a genetic disorder whose chromosome origins will shortly be unravelled.

symptoms and diagnosis

● As with neuroblastoma, the most common feature is a symptomless, painless abdominal mass, more commonly on the left and often discovered by the parent.
● Sometimes the child complains of passing discoloured, cloudy or blood-stained urine.
● Most of the other symptoms are less specific – lethargy, fever and poor appetite.
● Fewer than half of these children have secondary deposits at other sites when first examined, which is obviously good news from the point of view of curability. When the tumour does spread, it extends locally into the areas surrounding the kidney, to local lymph node groups, and, more distantly, to the lung (unlike the typical pattern in neuroblastoma), brain and bone. The opposite kidney may also be affected as a separate secondary site. Unlike neuroblastoma there are no well-recognised marker substances, but X-rays, CT, MRI and/or PET scanning, will define the extent of the primary tumour and presence of secondary deposits. These tests will also give the surgeon essential information as to the likely operability of the tumour at its primary site.

MOST COMMON SYMPTOMS OF WILMS' TUMOUR
Painless unilateral abdominal mass Sometimes cloudy or blood-stained urine Malaise Fever Poor appetite

treatment

Surgical removal is the most important goal of initial treatment, though chemotherapy is also highly effective, so much so that chemotherapy has become an important part of treatment even in early cases. This, again, is in contrast to the situation in neuroblastoma – in Wilms' tumour, chemotherapy is used for virtually every case. It is often given pre-operatively to shrink the tumour – the specifics of treatment will vary at different centres, though generally following national guidelines. The position of post-operative radiotherapy is also controversial. Its traditional role, i.e. in the treatment of children with an incomplete operation, and with involved local lymph nodes or tumour rupture during surgery, could be at an end since chemotherapy could turn out to be more beneficial, and less toxic than abdominal radiation.

prognosis   Children with Wilms' tumour generally do very well, and over three-quarters are cured. It's perfectly possible to live a fully normal life with only one kidney, of course. More difficult to cure are the bilateral cases – when both kidneys are involved – but the advent of more conservative surgical techniques and, where necessary, renal transplantation has greatly improved the outlook even for these difficult cases.

THE CHANCES OF INHERITING RETINOBLASTOMA

• Bilateral disease is almost always familial.

• Offspring survivors of hereditary retinoblastoma, or of bilateral sporadic cases, will have a 50% chance of developing the tumour.

• Unaffected parents with a child with unilateral disease have a 1 to 4% chance of having another affected child.

• Survivors of unilateral sporadic disease have a 7 to 10% chance of having an affected child, and are therefore presumed to be silent carriers.

• If two or more siblings are affected there is a 50% chance that subsequent siblings will have the tumour.

• Unaffected children from retinoblastoma families may occasionally (5%) carry the gene but if they have an affected child the risk in subsequent children is 50% since the parent is then identified as a silent carrier.

RETINOBLASTOMA

Retinoblastoma is a unique and often familial malignant tumour of the eye. The disease arises from the retinal layer, the pigmented, light-sensitive part at the back of the eye. Typically it spreads forwards, sometimes producing retinal detachment. The retina is the innermost layer of the eye, and extension backwards to the coating (the sclera) or optic nerve is unusual. More distant spread can occur either to the CSF or blood, sometimes producing secondary deposits in bone marrow, liver, lungs and other sites.

Retinoblastomas are rare, but are extremely important biologically, with a genetically determined familial incidence. The incidence has increased considerably over the past 40 years, the tumour now accounting for about 3% of all childhood cancers. The increasing incidence is due to increasing survival, leading to an increase in the number of children born to previously affected survivors, who have now become parents themselves.

The genetic pattern is complicated and despite the well-recognised family clustering, most cases of retinoblastoma are in fact sporadic (i.e. non-familial). In the genetic form, transmission is via a non-sexual (autosomal) dominant gene, meaning that offspring of survivors will have a 50% chance of developing the tumour themselves, since the term 'dominant' means that only one gene (of a pair) is necessary for the disease to become manifest – unlike the 'recessive' genetic illnesses in which both genes have to be faulty.

Non-familial cases are generally one sided (unilateral), with only a small risk (about 7 to 10%) that children of survivors will themselves be affected. Unaffected parents of a child who develops unilateral disease have a very small risk (under 5%) of having another affected child, but in rare cases where both eyes are affected – even without a background family history – there is a 50% chance that when they grow up, their children could develop the disease. A further important point is that in family cases, most of the affected children will unfortunately develop bilateral disease, so that, in an apparently unilateral case, very close watch must be kept on the opposite (contralateral) eye.

symptoms and diagnosis

● Most children affected by retinoblastoma develop it before the age of two, generally with a white pupil which can be quite noticeable and often picked up as an obvious difference between the two eyes (lack of the 'red eye' effect) when family photos are taken indoors with a flash camera. The difference is due to the inability of the affected eye to reflect light in the usual way, and the white pupil is sometimes termed a 'cat's eye reflex'.

● Later on, children with retinoblastoma often develop a squint, increased pressure in the eye (glaucoma) or difficulties with visual fixation (for example, with reading) or with vision generally.

● Total blindness is not a typical feature of retinoblastoma unless both eyes are grossly affected.

Early examination by the family doctor and referral to an eye specialist should lead to rapid diagnosis though, obviously, other diseases of the eye may be the cause of these worrying symptoms.

Once again, tumour staging gives an excellent guide as to the likely outcome, and for retinoblastoma, the stage depends on the number, position and size of the tumours within the eye. These features are permanently recorded by intra ocular photographic techniques both before and after treatment.

MOST COMMON SYMPTOMS OF RETINOBLASTOMA
Family history (in approximately 15% cases)   White pupillary reflex   Squint

treatment

It has now become much more possible to preserve the eye by use of radiotherapy, chemotherapy, photocoagulation or cryosurgery (local freezing) rather than removal of the affected eye itself. The radiotherapy techniques include not only external irradiation, but a highly sophisticated form of brachytherapy (see page 105) using radiation sources placed as closely as possible against the tumour site.

With single tumours above about 10 millimetres in size, external irradiation of the whole eye is frequently the treatment of choice and is often achievable with adequate preservation of vision, since the retina from which the tumour arises is much more tolerant of a high radiation dose than the lens and cornea at the front of the eye. These can usually be shielded out, without dangerously undertreating the important area. For all these reasons, treatment of retinoblastoma is a highly specialised field of oncology.

With more advanced cases, the child is obviously at greater risk of losing the eye, but even with bilateral cases, very good preservation of vision is often achieved. Fortunately, most retinoblastomas are sufficiently responsive to radiotherapy for only modest doses to be required, either of external beam or brachytherapy. If the radiation beam does have to pass through the lens, cataract formation may occur at a later stage, clouding the vision but fortunately reversible by lens extraction, where necessary.

One important potential long-term complication that is more troublesome, however, is the radiation-induced second tumour, particularly common in retinoblastoma and occurring in up to 10% of children (most frequently those who required repeated courses of radiotherapy to control recurrent or multiple tumours). This relatively high risk of second tumours reflects not only the dangers of radiotherapy, which for the most part are relatively minor, but also, for reasons that are not yet fully understood, a particular genetic predisposition to second cancers in patients with this disease.

prognosis

The results of treatment are extremely good, particularly in early cases where the cure rate (with normal or near-normal visual preservation) should be virtually 100%. Thankfully, it's now very unusual to have to remove the eye surgically. Cure rates of 75% are regularly achieved, even with more advanced cases.

For patients with high-risk tumours (i.e. those in whom cure is less certain), including those which have extended beyond the eye by the time of diagnosis, chemotherapy has been used, with partial success.

MOST COMMON SYMPTOMS OF RHABDOMYOSARCOMA

Painless mass at almost any site
In head and neck: protuberance, nasal obstruction

In urinary tract: urinary obstruction, bloodstained vaginal discharge
In limbs and trunk: painless mass

RHABDOMYOSARCOMA

The primary bone tumours of childhood are treated just as those of the older age groups (see pages 142-8), but there is one childhood soft tissue sarcoma that needs more discussion. This is the rhabdomyosarcoma, a tumour chiefly occurring in children between two and five years of age and with different microscopic features from the typical adult type. It accounts for 50% of all the childhood soft-tissue sarcomas.

symptoms and diagnosis

● In young children, the most common type generally develops as a painless mass at a variety of sites including trunk, limb and head and neck, and the eye-socket, a site at which protuberance of the eye itself will be the main clinical feature (an example is shown in the photographs opposite).
● These tumours can spread widely, both to lymph nodes and also more distantly, to the lungs and bone marrow.

As with all paediatric tumours, management guidelines are complicated and very dependent on tumour stage, which in turn is determined by the usual blood, X-ray and scanning tests. Progress in the management of this tumour has been very rapid over the past 20 years and continues to be made.

treatment

Chemotherapy is highly effective and is now given pre-operatively, after biopsy confirmation, with relatively conservative surgical resection, post-operative irradiation and chemotherapy within national study guidelines. In some cases, particularly the deeply situated tumours in the facial area, surgery isn't generally performed at all, in order to avoid unnecessary mutilation. Local irradiation and early (adjuvant) chemotherapy can be extremely successful, often achieving a cure with less in the way of long-term damage than if surgery were used as well.

prognosis

Although several of the currently used chemotherapy drugs are known to be valuable, new agents and more intensive dose schedules are under investigation, particularly for patients with secondary spread, since these are much more difficult to cure by conventional means. Nonetheless, the majority of children with this disease are cured, in sharp contrast to the situation up to 1975. In patients with local disease, the cure rate is over 80%, with younger children (under the age of about seven) doing particularly well.

For many childhood cancers, the disease is rapidly brought under control, the child feels and looks well, and the clinical picture may even become more dominated by treatment side-effects than the initial damage wrought by the tumour itself. As the acute anxiety about the initial diagnosis fades in response to treatment success, so the nausea, vomiting, hair loss and disruption of school and family life all place a great strain on both the child and the rest of the family too. Brothers and sisters may feel 'left out' because of all the attention necessarily focused on their sibling, and they often, of course, have fears of their own, which they're afraid to express. Looking ahead, the long-term side-effects of treatment may produce new problems, some previously referred to, such as intellectual and neurological impairment, growth defects, infertility and other hormone effects. The child should be monitored for side-effects of treatment. Secondary treatment, if necessary, is likely to bring up all the old anxieties, most parents and children recognising that the situation is still more difficult than it was before, since the initial treatment had proved insufficient.

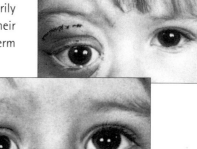

Fortunately, most of the childhood cancers can now be cured, the result of a remarkable sequence of research discoveries and collaboration, both at laboratory and clinical level. Studies of childhood cancer are often regarded as models to help in attempts at defining the most promising lines of attack in adult patients as well. With the advent of safer methods of supportive care, more intensive chemotherapy, and the recognition that most of the more common paediatric malignancies are responsive to treatment, there is every reason to hope that survival figures will continue to improve over the next decade.

This young child with a malignant tumour of the eye was treated with radiotherapy many years ago, before the advent of effective chemotherapy. Although he was cured, the orbit (eye socket) will never fully develop and the eyebrow will remain sparse. There is partial sight in the eye – but the left side is fine.

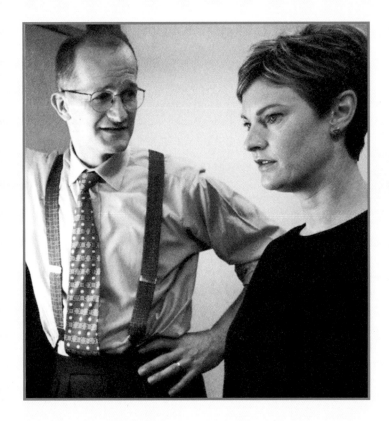

PART FOUR

INFORMATION AND SELF-HELP

❛ I've written down all my treatment
plans into three sections: mind, body,
spirit and I think all three of these
areas need to be tackled so that my
well-being is as strong as possible.❜

GLEN XAVIER

COMMON QUESTIONS AND ANSWERS

In the bad old days, the patient used to sit there silently, hardly daring to move or breathe – all the action came from behind the consultant's desk. It wasn't the patient's business to ask too many questions! Heavens, whatever next?

But all that has changed – or, at least it should have done. Patients have a right to know more about the treatment approaches that will affect them so profoundly: the benefits, side-effects, options, preferences – none of these are taboo subjects and for the doctor, exploration and discussion of these topics can all add up to one of the most gratifying parts of an otherwise humdrum working day.

Everyone must be aware, though – patients most particularly – that information is not only valuable but dangerous. In the search for reassurance, a patient with courage enough to ask, 'What's the chance of my being alive in a year's time?' may well receive a more gloomy response than expected – the moment's interchange altering forever his perception about his prospects and, in consequence, his priorities or choices for the future. Some relish the chance of proving the doctor wrong, others try to wish away the unwelcome news and need considerable extra support and more frequent follow-up visits.

Some of our most intelligent patients are, frankly, simply too worried about the potential side-effects of treatment for their own good. This is not to deny their right to know, but the doctor has to try to ensure that their understanding is well grounded within the proper context of the potential benefits and disadvantages of the treatment. There was, for example, a highly intelligent, 41-year-old journalist, mother of three young children, who read up all she could find about her tumour (including the medical textbooks), bombarded her consultant with literally dozens of written questions, mostly of the 'What if . . . ?' variety, attended for discussion at three or four hourly sessions, then finally refused the treatment that was clearly indicated. Less than two months later, despite a major operation (it was the radiotherapy she refused) the tumour had returned and – tragically too late – she now acquiesced to his original recommendation.

There comes a point where the patient, however bright, questioning and keen to retain control, has to invest his or her trust in the professional whose advice was sought in the first place. It's dispiriting, of course, for a consultant to take a grudging patient through treatments they would clearly prefer not to have, but far more tragic when the opportunity for a cure is lost, simply as a result of an unwillingness to recognise that the specialist is there to help, to be trusted. There are still too many patients in whom an initial opportunity for cure has passed because, for one reason or another, too little was done too late.

The following is a collection of the questions most commonly asked by cancer patients. The answers are not intended to be – and, indeed, cannot be – exhaustive, and they should not stop you from asking your own doctor and nurse for further information. Organisations listed in the Useful Addresses (see page 216) may also be able to answer queries.

Q/A

IS THERE ANYTHING I COULD HAVE DONE TO PREVENT THE CANCER?

In many cancers, there is only ever a very poor idea – sometimes no idea at all – as to what was the original cause or provocation. In brain tumours, cancers (sarcomas) of soft tissues such as muscle and cartilage, or glandular malignancies (lymphomas), virtually nothing is known about causation. No common thread has been found which defines the type of patient most likely to develop these, though there are plenty of fashionable, unsubstantiated theories to trap the unwary.

But, in an increasing number, oncologists really do have some idea (see pages 14-21). Lung cancer is, of course, the best example of all – the disease was pretty unusual before smoking became popular in the early part of this century. The link between smoking and most (but not all) forms of lung cancer is so tight that in most studies more than 90% of lung cancer patients have smoked, often heavily, at some time in their lives. In women who have never smoked but are married to smokers, the risk of their developing lung cancer is more than twice as great, compared with similar women who are married to non-smokers. Not surprising, perhaps – tobacco smoke contains over 4,000 different chemicals, many of which are known to be harmful. We now know that 50% of all cigarette smokers will die prematurely as a result of the habit – the most important single statistic to have emerged about the evils of tobacco.

Alcohol, too, can be dangerous, and is clearly a causative factor in the head and neck cancer group (see page 133). In populations with a high intake of meat, the risk of cancer of the large bowel is high, and there is now a general agreement that too much meat really is bad for you – eat more fibre! As for skin cancers; the advice is to avoid too much sun (discussed more fully on pages 127-8) . . . and so on.

The more we know about the causes of cancer, the more we can do to prevent their development. The current belief is that about 30% of all cancer deaths are caused by smoking and that a similar figure may be related to diet, though the evidence here is much less clear. But it will certainly help to eat more fruit and vegetables, less fatty foods and meat, and avoid too much alcohol. The Health Education Council issues an excellent, free booklet entitled *Cancer – How to Reduce Your Risks*, which gives further details.

So it's a complex question, particularly where there is a genetic component – such as breast cancer, where family history is probably the most powerful in a whole variety of contributing factors. You have to choose your parents with great care! But one myth that must be dispelled is that there is a specific type of 'cancer personality'. Much has been written about this, and it's all nonsense. It's so easy to imagine that 'It only happens to the best people' or 'He deserved what he got', but they are all meaningless, trivial phrases without any substance. We must have seen tens of thousands of patients with cancer, but there are no particular personality or emotional features in common. Contentions as important as this require scientific validation. It's all too easy for devotees of this or that culture to push their pet enthusiasm.

Cancer is often regarded as a stress-related illness, since so many patients give an account of major life events that have befallen them in the months preceding the diagnosis – a broken marriage, financial disaster, death of a loved one and so on. But ask almost anyone about the last year of their life, and you'll find that there'll usually be some dreadful item to relate.

Q/A

IS CANCER ALWAYS PAINFUL?

Uncontrolled pain is something people are very fearful of. Some cancers cause no physical pain. There are patients who have pain but there has been much progress in preventing or controlling pain.

It is very important that patients with advanced disease should be comfortable. It is advantageous to discuss with your doctor or nurse if you are experiencing pain so that something can be done to help relieve it. It may be necessary for a referral to be made to seek the advice of a pain specialist.

Q/A

SHOULD I CHANGE MY DIET/LIFESTYLE TO ENSURE THE CANCER DOESN'T RETURN?

This is a tricky one too. As far as diet is concerned, the general points outlined above are worth taking seriously. Try to cut down on fatty foods, meat (if you're an over-enthusiastic carnivore) and alcohol – not more than 21 units a week for men or 14 for women. With some cancers (the head and neck group, stomach, liver and pancreas), it might be better to give up altogether, since alcohol may well have played a part in their causation. In any event, many patients find it easier to cut out alcohol altogether than to cut it down and keep it at a more reasonable level. Smoking is obviously best avoided – though, paradoxically perhaps, it's not fair to bully certain patients about this too much – those with hopelessly incurable cancers, for example – particularly if smoking is one of their few remaining pleasures and to give up would be difficult. What's the point of stopping smoking for this unfortunate group? Sadly, it won't turn the clock back. But patients with cured head and neck cancer, for example, should be urged to stop smoking at all costs; it's a tragic fact that the most common cause of death in patients cured of an early cancer of the larynx is a new, separate, lung cancer from continued smoking – the very same cause that was responsible for the cancer of the larynx in the first place. Every radiotherapist in the country has lost patients this way, so be sensible, eat healthily, avoid too much sun, and, if exposed to dangerous substances at work, follow the precautions about protective clothing.

As far as lifestyle is concerned, there is no need to make much alteration here, just for the sake of it. 'Change of lifestyle' mostly means reducing your stress level – easier said than done. The trouble with paying too much attention to this concept is that it's so easy for the illness to become the focus of the patient's life – change the diet, add in the vitamins, alter the lifestyle and so on – often just taking a more robust attitude would be better.

You've finished the treatment? You're a few years on? Good! Why not forget your previous medical history altogether, or at least push it to the margins of your life, rather than letting it continue to occupy centre stage. You've got a life to live, after all. There are more important things to do than worry about whether or not the latest food fad or trace element theory might give you an extra per cent or two in your long-term chances. Remember that the food additive industry is a multi-billion-pound affair and that cancer patients are prime and highly susceptible targets. If you eat sensibly and well – plenty of fruit, vegetables and fresh food – you won't need any additives at all.

Q/A

HOW DO I TELL MY FAMILY/CHILDREN OR FRIENDS THAT I HAVE CANCER?

If you are concerned about this issue then speak to one of the health care team, who will be able to advise you. There are skilled professional staff such as counsellors or clinical nurse specialists who may be able to help or it may be useful to talk to someone who has been through a similar experience or to attend a support or self-help group.

Q/A

WILL TREATMENT MAKE ME INFERTILE?

Chemotherapy can certainly cause infertility, though not all the drugs do this. In young women, the risk is fairly small. On the whole, the younger the patient, the less likely she is to become infertile, presumably because the reserve store of eggs in the ovary is fixed, and the closer the patient is to her natural menopause, the more likely the chemotherapy is to completely interrupt the fertile period. Fortunately, not many women after the age of, say, 40 have a continuing wish to conceive – though this, of course, can be a real issue in clinical management decisions. Even high doses of chemotherapy (of the intensity often employed with bone marrow transplantation) can be compatible with a later pregnancy – a patient recently produced healthy twins after just such a procedure, having suffered for ten years beforehand with a relapsing form of Hodgkin's disease.

In the case of young women treated for breast cancer, the traditional view in the past was that they should be discouraged from ever becoming pregnant again, on the grounds that the oestrogen surge that occurs during pregnancy could be extremely damaging for them and provide just the kind of environment that the cancer would exploit, developing once again in the favourable milieu. On the whole, this view is no longer taken, at least not to the same level of absolute diktat, though it is probably best to caution women that there is a possible theoretical risk of this kind. On the whole, though, the scant evidence there is on the subject seems to be reassuring. Women who are desperate to become pregnant after treatment for breast cancer will obviously have to decide for themselves what their priorities are.

In men, chemotherapy can certainly cause infertility, the details again depending on the specifics of the drugs and the dosages used. Unlike the situation in women, however, it is perfectly possible to freeze sperm and use the sample later, to inseminate the wife or partner if it becomes clear, after successful treatment for the cancer, that the patient's fertility has been damaged beyond repair. In young men who have been treated for cancer, the issue of fertility should always be explored and sperm storage offered. But there is quite a lot of evidence that many men are cured of chemo-responsive cancers without suffering permanent sterility.

Radiotherapy is a different matter. There is no risk of infertility whatsoever, provided that the gonads (the ovaries or the testicles) aren't irradiated directly, except for a very small number of patients (generally children or adolescents) in whom a course of radiotherapy for a brain tumour may damage the pituitary area. Even in these patients, however, it is generally possible to deal adequately with the problem, through simple hormone replacement, if puberty (and therefore fertility) does not occur naturally.

If radiotherapy is a necessary part of treatment, either directly to the ovaries or both testes, there is virtually no prospect of continued fertility, because of the damage directly caused to the ova (eggs) or sperm precursors. This point also applies to the large majority of patients treated by total body irradiation – usually as an adjunct to bone marrow transplantation for leukaemia or other disorders.

When cancer patients do conceive and have children (or father them), the risks of damage to the developing foetus are very small indeed, probably negligible, as a result of the cancer treatment though we do, on the whole, suggest to patients that they try to ensure an 18 to 24-month period between the end of their treatment and any attempt to conceive.

Q/A

WILL TREATMENT AFFECT MY SEX LIFE?

Quite likely, initially. Obviously this is one of the most complex and sensitive of issues, but there are a number of important points to make. First, the news of the diagnosis itself, and the complicated psychological reactions afterwards – anger, bitterness, sadness, guilt, frustration and so on – are hardly conducive to nights of passion. This is an important point – partners have to be supportive, understanding and flexible. On the other hand, there are couples who find that the diagnosis of a life-threatening condition brings them closer in all respects (including sex), so it would be foolish to suggest hard-and-fast advice as to what might happen. As for the treatment itself, it's the sickness and debilitation and fatigue following a major operation, radiotherapy or chemotherapy that is more likely to reduce your libido, rather than the specific effects of, say, the chemotherapy agents themselves. If your sex life does suffer after treatment, it's not likely to be due to any organic treatment-related cause, but it's much more frequently a totally understandable psychological reaction to a highly threatening and anxiety-provoking experience. There is no reason why your sex life shouldn't return to normal afterwards, even if it has been somewhat affected during the treatment.

There are one or two caveats to this, chiefly concerning treatment by hormone therapy in men with prostate cancer. For example, radical operations can lead to impotence (though recent developments have meant that even a radical prostectomy need not always have this effect). The hormones that are often used in prostate cancer can render men impotent as well.

An equally important group for special mention includes younger women with gynaecological cancers or breast cancer, in whom treatment by surgery, radiation or chemotherapy has brought on an early menopause. Although this may be desirable, as, for example, in patients with breast cancer, the effects can be profound. Many patients complain bitterly about the early ageing, loss of skin, hair and general body tone and perhaps, especially, loss of libido, this latter often compounded by discomfort or bleeding during intercourse as a result of the thinning of the vaginal lining. In the case of patients with gynaecological cancers suffering these troublesome side-effects, hormone replacement therapy (HRT) is both safe and effective – a real life-saver in many.

On the whole, there seems no reason whatever to deny women HRT, apart from the small group of pre-menopausal patients with endometrial cancer in whom oestrogen replacement is generally regarded as undesirable, since it might stimulate regrowth of the cancer. Some specialists feel the same level of concern for patients with cancer of the cervix (neck of the womb) who have an adenocarcinoma (a glandular-type cancer), which mimics, at least in its appearance under the microscope, the cancers more typically associated with the lining of the womb. Even in this group, however, it is at least possible to use progestogen drugs, such as Provera or Megace, which often give a fair degree of recovery, even though they don't contain any oestrogen; a more recently available drug, known as Tibolone (Livial), can also be helpful in this respect.

Pre-menopausal patients with breast cancer present a particular problem since, increasingly, chemotherapy is used in this group, for very good reasons but with the side-effect of producing an early menopause. Since many surgeons and other specialists believe that the induction of the early menopause is a key part of the therapeutic effect, it seems illogical to use HRT for such patients, although the traditional view has softened a little in recent years. Once again, Provera, Livial or similar drugs can be extraordinarily valuable, without the potential dangers of HRT. In severe unresponding cases, a miserable life without HRT can be so dreadful for the patient, and possibly so disruptive to her marital and sexual relationships, that HRT should be used. Modest doses of Provera (around 20 milligrams a day) are effective in about two-thirds of all patients in reducing, or even abolishing, the menopausal effects – not bad for an agent that doesn't contain any oestrogen and seems perfectly safe both on practical and theoretical grounds.

Q/A

WHAT SHOULD I DO IF THE CANCER IS DIAGNOSED WHEN I AM PREGNANT, OR IF I CONCEIVE DURING TREATMENT?

Fortunately, this does not occur very often, and it's not really possible to give absolute guidance. Each individual case will depend very much on the circumstances. For example, in a woman of 32, with three healthy children, diagnosed with a potentially fatal yet curable gynae-cological cancer during the early stages of pregnancy, the strong advice of most specialists would be to allow treatment to proceed in order to cure the mother, even though this will inevitably result in termination of the pregnancy. In cancer of the cervix, for instance, where the cure rates are high if the disease is diagnosed and treated early, this must surely be the right advice. On the other hand, if the disease is diagnosed during the final stages of pregnancy, with delivery only a couple of months away, it is not so unreasonable, especially if the pregnancy is a particularly 'precious' one, to keep a very careful watch on the preg-nancy, induce labour or deliver by caesarian section at the earliest safe opportunity, and then get on quickly with the normal treatment within a short time afterwards.

With chemotherapy treatments, similar difficult decisions have to be made. Take the case of a very young woman with widespread breast cancer, six months pregnant and with only a small chance of surviving herself to the expected delivery date. Chemotherapy seemed the only possible means of keeping her alive, but might it harm the baby? The decision was to go ahead and treat her, since the obstetric advice was that the baby's organs would be fully formed already, and fortunately she gave birth to a healthy 8-pound boy just a few weeks before she herself died from this terrible disease.

It's sometimes possible, though specialists are never terribly happy about it, to give radiotherapy during pregnancy. Another patient was a young research scientist who, after many unsuccessful years, had final-ly become pregnant. Sadly, this coincided soon afterwards with a relapse of her previously diagnosed breast cancer. She developed sec-ondary deposits in her brain, causing partial paralysis and facial weak-ness. One specialist advised her to terminate the pregnancy in order to allow immediate treatment. Another felt that she should face the inevitability of this being a totally incurable situation – which, in her heart of hearts, she knew anyway. An immediate termination would not have turned an incurable disease into a curable one. Once she and her husband realised this, they were both adamant that the condition be treated as far as possible without a termination. Fortunately, her condition improved with steroids for the first six weeks, and radiotherapy to the brain was possible at a later stage without too much radiation dose scattering down to the pelvis (we checked this with dose monitors, of course). She, too, gave birth to a fine baby boy, and lived another four months or so.

Q/A

WILL MY HAIR FALL OUT? WILL IT TAKE YEARS TO GROW BACK?

Unfortunately, many chemotherapy drugs do cause hair loss (alopecia). Obviously the oncologist or nurse supervising your care will tell you how likely this is with the particular group of drugs that has been recommended for you. The major culprits include doxorubicin (Adriamycin), vincristine, etoposide, taxol and daunorubicin – there are several more. The good news is that it can be absolutely guaranteed that the hair loss will be temporary (there aren't many areas in cancer medicine where such an absolute guarantee can be made, so this really is quite a prize!) and that the quality of the hair, including colour, should be pretty similar to how it was previously. Quite often, the hair returns in a more 'youthful' condition – finer, silkier or more wavy. There have even been one or two partly bald men who ended up with more hair after chemotherapy than they had in the first place. It doesn't usually take all that long – there are many instances of patients regrowing hair even before completion of the chemotherapy administration. Within three months or so, hair regrowth should be very satisfactory. We recognise that it can be upsetting to lose your hair temporarily. Sometimes we can try to reduce hair loss by using 'scalp cooling'. This means wearing a cold cap on your head for about two hours at the time of your chemotherapy administration. It is not effective for all chemotherapy regimes but your chemotherapy nurse can advise if it would be suitable for use in your situation.

Radiotherapy also affects the hair, but only when the radiation beam is directed at the skull – generally for a primary or secondary brain tumour (see page 173). It is surprising how many people believe that radiotherapy can cause hair loss on the scalp, even when it has been given to a distant part of the body – chest, abdomen or pelvis. This is simply not so.

Hair recovery after radiotherapy is a more uncertain and generally slower affair than after chemotherapy. It is highly dose dependent, i.e. recovery will be much quicker after a small dose than a very large one. There are many instances where, sadly, hair regrowth is poor, even after several years, particularly at the top of the head where the radiation beam passes across the top of the skull almost tangentially, creating pockets of high dosage, which are impossible to avoid. Life for the radiotherapist would be much easier if the skull were shaped like a sugar-cube!

It is generally possible to mask these difficulties if there really is troublesome delay of hair regrowth, either by hair pieces or, more simply, by adjusting the hair style so that the uncovered areas are disguised. A very few patients feel so psychologically damaged, though, that they request a referral to a plastic surgeon or hair expert. There are one or two cunning techniques available, including hair transplantation or the use of an expandable device which the surgeon can fit under the hair-bearing area of the scalp, gradually increasing the volume, so that a dome of hair-bearing skin develops on the patient's scalp – some of this redundant flap then being used as a hair-bearing skin graft to cover the defective site.

Although these techniques are in common use elsewhere, particularly in the USA, there (fortunately) doesn't seem to be too much demand in this country. Most patients simply learn to cope – and, in any event, life is rather easier these days, since a much wider range of hair styles, including very close cropping and partial baldness, are now considered socially acceptable.

Q/A

WITH ME HAVING HAD CANCER, ARE MY CHILDREN MORE AT RISK?

On the whole, the answer to this is an unequivocal 'no'. There are very few cancers with such a strong genetic component that children will be at high risk. Perhaps the best known is the very rare childhood cancer of the eye, known as retinoblastoma, in which the genetics are very well understood; this is discussed fully on pages 188-9. A much more common problem, however, is the patient with breast cancer – itself a familial disease, of course – who has a strong family history of the disease. There is no doubt that daughters of patients with breast cancer are at greater risk of developing the disease (probably about double) and that the more family members affected, the more likely the risk. No one quite knows what to do with this information, and, in the USA, the operation of bilateral prophylactic subcapsular mastectomy (i.e. removal of both breasts before there is any sign of disease, but with preservation of the skin and nipples, together with immediate reconstruction) has become a little more popular in recent years in women from high-risk families who request it.

This very drastic approach has not yet taken hold in the UK or Europe, but one can understand both the ghastly logic and the terrible predicament of a young woman who knows that she is at very high risk by virtue of a strong family history. It's probably sensible for such patients to be screened at a genetic or breast family history clinic from an earlier age (mid-30s, say, rather than the normal recommendation of 50 years) using mammography, which should be repeated every two years or so.

Other familial cancer syndromes are very unusual. There is a type of familial bowel disorder, characterised by multiple polyps which have a high propensity to malignant change, and, once again, screening is generally recommended for these patients, using direct vision by colonoscopy (see also page 111).

Families with a high incidence of ovarian cancer are also well recognised. On the whole, though, the genetic component of cancer is not sufficiently strong to represent a real threat to any offspring of cancer patients. The best advice, of course, is: don't smoke, eat sensibly, avoid too much sunlight.

Q/A

CAN WE BE SURE THE
CANCER IS GONE?

All cancers are different, and some are particularly unpredictable, capable of reappearing unexpectedly after many years when all traces had apparently been eradicated. The good news, though, is that these are less common than the large numbers in which, after five years free of recurrence of disease, one can be pretty certain that the disease will not recur. This applies to the large bulk of cancers we treat, and in a small number, one can even be pretty confident after as little as two or three years. Testicular tumours, for example, were so vicious before today's effective treatments that they would generally reappear (if they were going to come back at all) within two years or so. With modern treatment, freedom from recurrence for a two-year period is virtually tantamount to cure. The same applies for the small-cell variety of lung cancer (the type which is most closely associated with smoking), which is so malignant that recurrence after treatment is very common within two years, only a small minority of patients proving to be cured in the long run. In head and neck cancer sites, the two- or three-year rule applies once again: relapses after this time are uncommon, and follow-up visits to the clinic won't have to be so frequent, most specialists insisting on a monthly follow-up schedule during the crucial first year, which represents the real danger period.

The major exception to all this is breast cancer, which is a dreadfully capricious disease, capable of lying quiescent for ten years or more, then returning quite unexpectedly. Although this might sound like an impossible, Damoclean situation, the very late relapse of this type is fortunately uncommon. Over two-thirds of breast cancer patients remain alive and well during the first five years of treatment, the majority of whom will remain disease-free at the tenth year of follow-up as well. Other conditions where relapses can occur late include melanoma and cancer of the kidney, which can also behave in a very curious way. It can apparently remain under total control, without evidence of residual disease, but then late relapse can occur – a very well-documented occasional feature.

For all these reasons, it's difficult to generalise, but, in most cases, freedom from disease at, say, the five-year mark is pretty good evidence of cure. Follow-up clinics are extremely important; they not only help the specialist to build up an ever more complete picture of you (and perhaps your family as well), but also provide excellent opportunities for training young doctors and nurses who hope to become specialists themselves as well as the medical students who so badly need to know that cancer patients can indeed lead active, fruitful and often untroubled lives after treatment. From the patient's point of view, of course, they represent an important part of the insurance against recurrence, or at least the early recognition of recurrent disease with, hopefully, some prospect of further active treatment.

Q/A

WHAT HAPPENS IF THE CANCER COMES BACK?

There is an important difference between recurrence at the initial, or primary, site and recurrence at a distant site or sites (secondary deposits). With recurrence at the primary site, it is sometimes possible to operate again, to remove the whole of the diseased area – or to offer radiotherapy, if this has not previously been done. Patients with brain tumours, cancers of the large bowel recurring at the site of the area where the two cut ends of the bowel had been joined together again after the first operation to remove the tumour and breast cancer quite often fall into this group. For many breast cancer patients these days, in whom a small local excision operation has been followed by radiotherapy, recurrence at the primary site (which occurs in about 7% of such patients) can be managed very successfully, though this usually means a mastectomy, or, at the very least, a wider operation than was originally performed. If, for technical reasons, surgery is no longer possible, then radiotherapy is often useful, provided it hasn't already been given to this same area.

Where the recurrence is of the rather more common secondary type, at distant sites or in local lymph node (glandular) areas, the ball game is altogether different. Local lymph node spread can sometimes be dealt with surgically, but, in general, patients with this type of recurrence are very difficult to cure. For most cancers, it isn't the primary but the secondary deposits, with their often relentless pattern of spread, that prove fatal in the end. Chemotherapy or hormone therapy are often well worthwhile, however, since they can both help to halt the progress of the secondaries. Very occasionally it is still possible to cure patients, even at this late stage – testicular and thyroid cancers are good examples, discussed more fully on pages 124 and 139-40.

Since chemotherapy can be quite a troublesome form of treatment for the patient, it can be difficult to decide whether events should be allowed to take their course, so to speak, or perhaps to take a more active line and offer chemotherapy, even in unpromising circumstances. This difficult judgement is usually best made by careful discussion with the patient, sometimes with the family as well, and deciding together what seems best. The patient certainly shouldn't be under any illusions as to what can reasonably be expected, but palliative treatment of this kind can be extremely valuable in reducing symptoms and perhaps granting the patient a few extra months or even years. Sometimes one is pleasantly surprised even in unpromising circumstances. Hormone therapies can be extremely valuable as well, though perhaps for a more limited group of diseases – cancers of the breast, prostate and uterus are the best examples. All of these may prove responsive, even if spread to distant sites has occurred, for periods of months or even years, generally with few side-effects. It is for this reason that most specialists still prefer to use hormone therapy first, before chemotherapy, in diseases such as breast cancer where either could reasonably be offered.

If the opportunity for active treatment really has passed, most patients (but not all – there aren't any hard-and-fast rules) prefer to know rather than be fobbed off. The doctor's responsibility doesn't end here, of course. A good oncologist should always be prepared to stay with the patient until the end along with other health care professionals often in conjunction with a Community Palliative Care Team or Macmillan nurse, offering support, counselling and – perhaps most important of all – the practical advice, which can be of such great help. Symptom control has advanced so much in recent years that very few patients are unresponsive to the right kind of symptom control – an enormous subject, covered more fully on pages 64-5.

Q/A

If you are worried about finances or not being able to manage, then ask to see a benefits advisor or social worker who will offer advice. Your local Citizens Advice Bureau is another useful source of information.

WHAT HELP CAN SOCIAL SERVICES PROVIDE?

Q/A

Internal surgery should not make any difference at all, apart from the scar, of course. Some of the most exciting advances in cancer surgery over the past decade have been based not only on technical improvements, but also on the increasing recognition that body image really is important – hence the emphasis on local excision with breast preservation, rather than mastectomy, if at all possible. Breast reconstruction is, of course, a real option for patients who are keen to have it. Surgeons vary as to the techniques they use and when they feel it should best be performed, but in general, far more women are now opting to at least explore the possibility of a breast reconstruction, which can sometimes include the nipple as well. For the most part, recent scares about leakage of silicone implants seem largely without foundation, and some of the really sophisticated techniques don't rely on these implants so heavily, anyway. In malignant bone tumours, particularly those affecting the limbs in young adolescents, advances in conservative and restorative surgery have been really astonishing. Even as little as 20 years ago, amputation was almost always required, whereas we now

WILL MY PHYSICAL APPEARANCE BE AFFECTED BY TREATMENT?

have a whole series of bio-engineered, tailor-made internal metallic implants, some of which even have expandable shafts for growth, which allow preservation of the adult or growing limb.

Even facial operations can often be achieved with a minimum of external scarring and deformity, since surgeons are often very expert at devising their operations to allow placement of the surgical scar in a natural fold of skin – a forehead crease or the crease which runs down the side of the nose, for example. But, of course, it should be recognised that altered body image can be very distressing for the patient and often a scar, however small, is a permanent reminder of the causes of its treatment. Laryngectomy leaves a permanent stoma (hole) at the front of the neck, but this is usually disguised by a small pad that is porous enough to allow for breathing (that's the point of the stoma, of course), and a collar and tie or high neck-line will often disguise most of this, anyway. Speaking valves are also more widely used nowadays. Recent advances in plastic surgery and in facial prostheses can give people a better cosmetic appearance.

The issue of hair loss from radiotherapy and chemotherapy has already been discussed on page 48. In other respects, neither of these treatments should cause permanent scarring or change of body image, though high doses of radiotherapy can sometimes lead to subtle skin changes, which may be permanently visible – small leashes of tiny veins, or areas of additional or deficient pigmentation. On the whole, these shouldn't be too marked with normal radiation techniques – unless, of course, the site has to be re-irradiated because of local recurrence, though radiotherapists are always very cautious about this. Radiotherapy can also lead to permanent loss of body hair in the site irradiated (armpit, pubic area, chest and so on), though very few patients are at all concerned about this.

Q/A

CAN I ASK FOR A SECOND OPINION FROM ANOTHER CANCER SPECIALIST?

Of course you can! It is perfectly reasonable for patients with cancer who have several options for treatment of their disease to seek a second opinion. In the first instance, it is wise to discuss this issue with your specialist or with your general practitioner.

Q/A

THE ONCOLOGIST TELLS ME IT'S A 'LOW-GRADE' TUMOUR, SO I SHOULDN'T WORRY TOO MUCH. WHAT ON EARTH'S HE TALKING ABOUT?

This is quite a common question. Tumour grading is a term used to describe the inherent growth characteristics of cancers; this is done by careful microscopic examination in the pathology lab of the tissue, which was removed or sampled by biopsy. Under the microscope, low-grade tumours sometimes appear not all that different from the normal tissues they arise from, whereas the higher-grade cancers look much more disordered, even bizarre. Most tumours show characteristics of either low, intermediate or high grade, a single variety rather than a jumble; though, of course, there can be exceptions to this general rule.

The importance of grading is that the clinician in charge of a patient can use the information to help assess the severity of each case and, to some extent, predict both its likely speed of evolution and general clinical behaviour. Low-grade tumours are often much more indolent than the higher grades: non-Hodgkin's lymphomas and brain tumours are good examples (see pages 153 and 168). For these tumours, pathological grade largely determines the choice of treatment. Low-grade lymphoma, for instance, may not require treatment at all (at least in the initial stages, which may last for many years, even after a firm diagnosis has been made), whereas high-grade lymphoma in a young, fit person inevitably requires combination chemotherapy and sometimes even a bone marrow transplant with intensive drug treatment and total body irradiation.

Q/A

DO ALL CHEMOTHERAPY DRUGS HAVE THE SAME SIDE-EFFECTS?

Sometimes people believe that all chemotherapy treatments are the same. But there are approximately 50 anti-cancer drugs in use today, which can be used in different, varying combinations depending on the type of cancer.

Each drug has different side-effects and these will be explained to you by your doctor and by the nurse who administers the treatment. Some side-effects may be hard to cope with while others will be mild (see page 48). Remember that not all chemotherapy causes nausea and hair loss. If the side-effects such as nausea are severe, there are drugs that are effective in controlling the problem.

Q/A

HOW WILL I FEEL MENTALLY AND EMOTIONALLY DURING THE TREATMENT?

Every patient reacts differently. For some, it's business as usual, all the way through. Others, on the other hand, find the whole business of diagnosis and treatment so distressing that the utmost reassurance and support seem to make little impact. For the most part, patients seem to cope remarkably well – possibly because the initial diagnosis is so upsetting that the knowledge that treatment is indeed available, coupled with the concern and professional expertise of the staff, is itself extremely therapeutic. Some years ago, a research team looking at breast cancer patients found that they could roughly divide them into four groups: those with 'fighting spirit', who mentally and physically rose to the challenge, so to speak; then at the other end of the emotional spectrum were those who were 'stoic acceptors' of the illness; in between was the 'helpless, hopeless' group, and finally the 'deniers', who put the whole affair to one side, as it were, and simply dismissed it in order to get on with their lives.

Although the work has remained controversial, it's always struck a chord, since many oncologists would recognise these responses. The really contentious part of the research was the suggestion that the personality characteristics might have a bearing on outcome, since two of these groups of patients seemed to do far better than the others. Interestingly, it was the first and last groups (those who deny and those with fighting spirit) who did well, the others much less so. Not perhaps what one might have expected, though quite what one makes of this research is not at all clear – it's no easy matter to change one's emotional responses, let alone one's personality!

Most patients feel well supported during the treatment itself, particularly since so many of the unpleasant, treatment-related symptoms can now be dealt with quite effectively by anti-nauseants, attention to skin care and so on. It is often much more difficult in the first weeks following completion of treatment, as if the sudden transition from intensive activity and clinic visits to a far more detached follow-up protocol is akin to being cast adrift on a choppy sea. Depression and anxiety are probably far more common during this period than during the treatment itself, often totally unrecognised both by the medical staff and the patient's family. What often makes it worse is that the patient often feels so guilty at this point – just at the time when champagne corks should be popping, he may possibly feel at his lowest ebb. Families and loved ones need to be particularly aware of this to avoid falling into the 'After all they've done for you . . . It's time to snap out of it' scenario. The truth, of course, is that the process of rehabilitation and re-entry into a normal lifestyle is only just beginning.

Q/A

WILL I BE ABLE TO CONTINUE WORKING DURING TREATMENT?

Tricky one, this. On the whole, yes. Strange to say, most people actually seem to enjoy their work – some even find it quite therapeutic to continue or resume normal activities, so to speak, rather than sit around at home, frustrated, bored and introspective. For many of us, work provides not only a degree of satisfaction, but also self-esteem – and the support of colleagues who provide, at the very least, a reminder of normality and may sometimes have been through the same thing themselves. The traditional view of enforced rest from work as an essential part of recovery has largely gone by the board, though obviously circumstances will vary.

Some types of work are physically too strenuous for a weakened patient to cope with, and some, such as teaching, may be too exposed or demanding; the ideal, perhaps, is a flexible arrangement whereby the patient can go in part time, or perhaps take a few weeks or months off entirely, before resuming part time in the first instance. In really high-pressure jobs, it may be best to withdraw entirely – a medical colleague, a consultant surgeon with cancer, told me that he found it extremely odd not to get up at 6.30 a.m. every day and be in the operating theatre by 7.45 a.m., and had real difficulty during the first fortnight dealing with his feelings of guilt and lowered self-esteem. After that, however, he saw it quite differently as the opportunity of a lifetime! It certainly makes many re-think their work patterns, and although the majority wish to resume as normal, some patients see their professional or working lives in a totally new perspective.

Most forms of cancer treatment are tiring – particularly, perhaps, an extended course of radiotherapy. You shouldn't underestimate this – it can be a potent cause of irritability and disenchantment if you attempt to return at full tilt too soon. Perhaps the hardest part is to recognise just how much you're capable of, pace yourself a bit, but don't expect yourself to perform at full capacity straight away. The tendency is to prove to the world that you're absolutely back to normal in record time – try to resist!

Q/A

WHAT ARE MY CHANCES OF SURVIVAL, AND MAKING A FULL RECOVERY?

Every patient has the right to ask this, though not all wish to. Not everybody wants to put the doctor on the spot, so to speak, or to risk hearing an unwelcome reply. As mentioned earlier in the book, a difficult situation can arise when a patient chooses not to ask this highly charged question him or herself but their spouse or partner does it for them, leaving the oncologist uncertain as to whether the patient would wish to voice the question at all. There is something rather improper about responding, unless it is clear that the patient (not just the spouse or companion) really does want to have the information.

In Part Three we have tried to give a reasonable account of the prospects for recovery for most of the main types of cancer, and there certainly isn't space here to recapitulate fully. However, for cancers that have remained localised at their point of origin, and are generally surgically removable or successfully treatable by radiotherapy, the chances of recovery are often high – over 90%, for example, in the case of a small cancer of the larynx treated by radiotherapy, with full preservation of the normal voice and powers of speech. In other cancers, with a higher tendency for spread, the outlook is obviously less certain, but even in these, modern research has increasingly provided methods for recognising the potential for tumour dissemination and, to some extent, pre-empting it – breast cancer is probably the best example, in which both chemotherapy and hormone treatments can be used prophylactically to lower the risk of this occurring.

It is now recognised that this can also be achieved, to some extent, with another large group of tumours – the colorectal (large bowel) cancers. The likelihood of recovery is determined not only by the details of anatomic sites of disease (the tumour stage), but also, as mentioned above, the pathological characteristics (tumour grade), as well as other factors, such as the chromosomal content of the malignant cells, the molecular cell markers, which can be determined by special staining methods in the laboratory, and the presence of tumour extension to local lymph node groups. All these points are both important and predictive of the outcome, yet we still fall far short of the ideal – an accurate determination of the prognosis for each patient, which at the very least would allow us to tailor our intensity of treatment with much greater confidence. For some tumours, particularly those that are chemo-sensitive, the completeness of the chemotherapy response is so important as a predictive factor for outcome that it may outweigh all other considerations – an observation which has led some oncologists to the conclusion that winding up the dose of chemotherapy might represent the most promising form of novel cancer therapy for partly responsive tumours. Quite a number of trial groups are investigating this at present.

Q/A

I'VE HEARD THE EXPRESSION THAT CLINICAL TRIALS ARE GOOD FOR YOU. CAN YOU EXPLAIN WHAT THIS MEANS?

There are various levels of reliability in medical data and information. First, at the lowest level, there is the clinicial anecdote – the individual patient story so beloved of tabloid newspapers, of the 'My grandfather smoked 70 cigarettes a day and lived to be 92 years old' variety. Then there are the small group studies, where a small group of patients are treated in a similar way and reported in the medical literature as 'clinical experience'. This, of course, is a major step forward from the clinical anecdote, since it implies a genuine spirit of inquiry on the part of the investigator, and an attempt to be consistent with respect to a novel treatment. And then there are the prospectively controlled randomised studies, which are far and away the most reliable means of detecting a genuine advance. The fundamental point is that most important principle of all scientific experiments (as every A-level science student learns) in that every detail of such an experiment should be held constant, with a single difference between the two study groups. This means that, if there is a genuine and reproducible difference in outcome, it must, as far as we can possibly tell, be due to that one variable.

Clinical trials really are good for you in that they ensure that you are treated to the highest possible standards of care. They also allow you to make a genuine contribution, which may benefit not only yourself, but also many others, and they ensure that the results of your treatment will be carefully documented and analysed. Regrettably this is not by any means the rule in non-trial situations. Most clinical trials are held together by an enthusiastic working party and a trial co-ordinator who travels around the country to the various centres ensuring that data are kept absolutely up to date and ready for proper statistical analysis. The importance of controlled clinical trials in cancer cannot be overemphasised, and they have certainly proven immensely influential, increasingly taken up by the media and rapidly disseminated, provided the quality of data is strong enough. All of us in the health service have become accustomed to the concept of auditing our treatment outcomes and, in my view, the controlled clinical trial is the best possible form of medical audit.

Patients with cancer should always ask their specialist whether there are any clinical trials currently taking place in his or her department (or nationally, to which he or she might be a contributing clinician) so that they can decide whether or not they wish to participate. If 'patient power' means anything at all, it surely means providing an opportunity for patients to ask questions, to be pro-active, to recognise that it is their life and not the clinician's that is at stake, and to seek the best possible standard of care.

Q/A

CAN ALTERNATIVE THERAPIES BE USED IN ADDITION TO MORE CONVENTIONAL TREATMENTS?

Most of the few really well-designed studies that have been performed have turned out negative (or, worse still, suggested that the unconventional treatment might possibly do harm). No evidence of anti-tumour activity has ever been presented in a convincing way, no evaluation of results or independent critical assessment of data has been given. The anecdotes offered are on the lowest level of clinical value (see above) and are often explicable by simple means. Some cancer patients who profess to have been cured by unconventional remedies have, in fact, been following a conventional path as well, so any claim for the value of the alternative therapy is clouded by a conventional treatment, which is likely to have been responsible for the benefit. In one of the few controlled studies of alternative cancer treatment, laetrile, a 'harmless yet effective' remedy approved by most alternative cancer 'authorities' was found to be entirely without benefit and yet with significant side-effects when assessed in over 500 cancer patients treated at the Mayo Clinic. At least one major multicentre study carried out more recently has confirmed that other similar claims have no factual basis.

There is also the potential problem that considerable sums of money can so easily be made from vulnerable, gullible and trusting patients. Of course, every cancer patient's wish is not only to get well again, but better still to make a contribution to his or her own recovery. But devoutly wishing something were true doesn't, alas, make it happen, and much harm, as well as the undoubted benefit from, say, a balanced, healthy diet, can be done by some of the unwise (but perhaps well-intentioned) suggestions that are made.

One of the many reasons that patients seek these remedies is a dissatisfaction with conventional medicine or with the doctor, which is a loss of faith and trust that must certainly be taken seriously. Doctors are certainly at fault – and must shoulder some of the responsibility – if patients cannot get sufficient of their time or reasonable answers to their questions. Patients often say that they tried alternative methods of treatment because they were given no hope or emotional support, because they found the prospect of radiotherapy or chemotherapy unnatural, because there was inadequate explanation and reassurance and because treatment was being unreasonably or thoughtlessly prolonged or aggressive, without any hint of benefit. If a patient does decide to discontinue treatment, against the advice of the specialists, it is, of course, only proper to advise the patient of what the consequences might be, but cruel to bully or browbeat the patient into continuing. The patient should at the very least be reassured that he or she would be welcome back at any later stage. Despite these harsh words it can be helpful to send a patient with cancer to a homeopath or other 'alternative' specialists. Many patients do have a mystical belief that a change of diet or lifestyle, or a visit to a herbalist or acupuncturist will generally be beneficial. Homeopathic physicians can have considerable rapport and communication skills in addition to their excellent doctoring skills. Perhaps this is the appeal of alternative medicine and also, incidentally, helps to explain why there isn't the swell of patients asking for referral that were so much a feature of the 1980s. With the much greater use of counsellors within the health service, and a higher level of understanding among doctors of the importance of communication, it seems the demand has considerably dwindled.

However, more and more patients are having complementary therapies alongside conventional medical care. It is complementary to medical treatment, not excluding it, and such techniques include relaxation therapies, visualization, homeopathy, aromatherapy and healing. Many patients have found that these therapies have helped them during their cancer treatment. Studies have shown that acupuncture can reduce the nausea after chemotherapy. It can also sometimes be helpful in pain relief and in help with fatigue by boosting energy levels.

It is a good idea to inform your doctor if you are using a complementary therapy. For instance, aromatherapy should not be used on the skin of the area of body that is being treated by radiotherapy.

summary

All specialists are busy, sometimes rushed off their feet, but most are only too willing to try to answer questions. Do be ready with them, though – the amount of time available will inevitably be limited, and you will naturally want to use it in the best possible way. You will be treated by a team of specialist health care professionals: specialist nurses, chemotherapy nurses and radiographers. So do talk to them if you have any queries or need a question answered.

There is no point in pretending, though, that one can predict the future with complete accuracy, so don't be surprised if some of the replies are somewhat guarded. Living with uncertainty may be the most difficult part of the whole illness, but facing up to both the facts and the limitations of what is known is undoubtedly the best means of regaining some sort of control over your affairs. Good luck!

GLOSSARY OF DRUGS IN CANCER TREATMENT

This is not an exhaustive list of drugs but the agents mentioned are all well established in clinical use. There are many newer treatments still under investigation.

Anastrazole (Arimidex) Potent anti-oestrogen hormone used for breast cancer. An agent with a big future.

Aspirin Non-steroidal anti-inflammatory drug to deal with mild or moderate pain.

Bleomycin Agent widely used for testicular, head and neck as well as some of the pelvic and lung cancers.

Busulfan Drug used in treatment of leukaemia.

Carboplatin Important cisplatin derivative with fewer side-effects than the parent compound.

Chlorambucil A tablet form of chemotherapy, often used in low-grade lymphoma.

Cisplatin One of the most important chemotherapy drugs, very widely used in testicular, ovarian, head and neck and other cancers. Intravenous only.

CMF Standard drug regimen used in the treatment of breast cancer (see cyclophosphamide, methodrexate and fluorouracil).

Co-codamol Analgesic for mild or moderate pain.

Codeine Drug for stronger pain relief; best used in conjunction with a laxative.

Co-dydramol Analgesic for mild or moderate pain.

Co-proxamol (Distalgesic) Analgesic to deal with mild or moderate pain.

Cyclophosphamide Chemotherapy drug used in treatment of breast cancer (see CMF).

Cyproterone Anti-androgen agent widely used in the treatment of prostate cancer.

Dexamethasone A potent steroid drug widely used for brain tumours; also for chemotherapy-induced nausea.

Diamorphine hydrochloride Opiate used in severe pain. Extremely valuable.

Diclofenac (Voltarol) Anti-inflammatory agent used for moderate pain.

Dihydrocodeine (DF118) Drug for stronger pain relief (codeine derivative); best used in conjunction with a laxative, as very constipating.

Domperidone Anti-nausea drug.

Doxorubicin (Adriamycin) Chemotherapy drug, with a wide spectrum of activity. Toxic to the heart in high dosage.

Etoposide Chemotherapy drug used in treatment of testicular cancer, small-cell lung cancers and others.

Fluorouracil Drug used in treatment of breast cancer (see CMF), large bowel cancer and many other indications. An anti-metabolite.

Goserelin Drug for long-term palliation and symptom control of prostate cancer. Also used in some breast cancer patients.

Granisetron Anti-nausea drug widely used for chemotherapy side-effects.

Hydroxyurea Drug used for some types of leukaemia.

Ibuprofen Anti-inflammatory agent.

Interferon Drug used in treatment of melanoma, myeloma, and chronic myeloid leukaemia.

Irinotecan Newer drug used for large-bowel cancers.

Melphalan Chemotherapy drug; can be given by mouth.

Methotrexate Chemotherapy drug used in treatment of breast cancer (see CMF), leukaemia, and other sites.

Mitomycin C Useful chemotherapy drug, often used as a radiosensitiser.

Morphine Strong opiate drug.

Naproxen (Naprosyn) Non-steroidal anti-inflammatory drug to deal with mild or moderate pain.

Nitrogen mustard (mustine) Chemotherapy drug; a toxic agent but with impressive activity in lymphoma and certain types of solid cancer.

Ondansetron Anti-nausea drug widely used for chemotherapy side-effects.

Oxaliplatin Newer platinum-derivative drug used in metastatic large-bowel cancer.

Paracetamol Very valuable for mild to moderate pain.

Prednisone A form of steroid therapy very widely used.

Progesterone A female hormone preparation, used in breast cancer and uterine treatment.

STI-571 (Glivec) Oral tyrosine kinase inhibitor – may well transform treatment of chronic myeloid leukaemia.

Tamoxifen Highly active anti-oestrogen drug effective for breast cancer.

Taxotere Important taxane agent used to treat several types of cancer.

Thalidomide After a disastrous start, this drug is now finding a useful role, e.g. for drug-resistant myeloma.

Taxol Semi-natural chemotherapy drug, initially synthesised from the yew tree. One of the taxane group.

Vincristine Widely used agent, a 'spindle-cell poison' capable of stopping cancer cell division. Other similar agents: vinblastine, vindesine.

GLOSSARY OF TECHNICAL TERMS

Adenocarcinoma A type of cancer in which the cellular origin is from glandular tissue.

Adjuvant systemic therapy Treatments such as chemotherapy or hormones, given shortly after completion of initial surgery or radiation therapy to the 'primary site' of the cancer. Its aim is to reduce the risk of the cancer spreading to produce secondary growth or 'metastases'.

AFP Alpha fetoprotein. A tumour marker substance produced by malignant tissue, often denoting testicular cancer but also raised in primary cancer of the liver. Detectable as a blood test. Extremely useful for following the progress of the patient's response to treatment.

Allogeneic bone marrow transplantation Transplantation of matched bone marrow from a donor – generally a sibling, though sometimes from a matched unrelated donor.

Alopecia Hair loss. Often results from chemotherapy but if so, the hair virtually always re-grows. If due to irradiation of the brain, the hair loss is often much more prolonged.

ALL Acute lymphoblastic leukaemia. A form of leukaemia, the most common childhood type; this is a disease of the lymphocytic white cell series.

AML Acute myeloblastic leukaemia. A type of acute leukaemia far less common in childhood; occurs more frequently in adults; a disease of the myeloid white cell line in the marrow.

Anorexia Loss of appetite.

Apoptosis Programmed cell death.

Ascites Malignant abdominal fluid, often causing obvious swelling or distension.

Autologous bone marrow transplantation Removal of part of the patient's own bone marrow before very high-dose chemotherapy; then returned to the patient's body to reduce the effects of the chemo-induced fall in blood count.

Axillary node dissection Removal of glands from the armpit area. A very common part of surgical management of breast cancer.

BCG *Bacelle Calmette Géurin.* An agent instilled into the bladder to slow down the rate of cancer growth in the bladder lining. Sometimes used in other cancers as well, such as melanoma.

Brachytherapy A form of radiation in which a radioactive wire or tube is placed directly against a tumour. Often used in accessible cancers such as cervix, tongue or lip. Increasingly used in oesophagus and lung. Sometimes the radioactive wires are passed deep into the tumour itself.

Bronchoscopy A technique for inspecting and taking biopsies of the main air-passages (bronchi) leading to the lungs. Used extensively in the diagnosis of lung cancer, under a light anaesthetic.

Calcitonin A tumour-marker substance usually elevated in the bloodstream in patients likely to develop a medullary carcinoma of the thyroid. Useful as an investigation of relatives of such patients as this can be a familial condition.

CEA Carcino-embryonic antigen. A tumour marker detectable by a blood test and often raised in patients with colonic or rectal carcinomas. Not as specific as some other blood tests.

Carcinogenesis The chain of events leading towards malignant change. A substance such as cigarette smoke, which initiates this process, is termed carcinogenic.

Carcinoma A malignant tumour originating from an organ with a surface, e.g. skin, tongue, bladder, rectum, prostate.

Chemosensitive A tumour that is responsive to chemotherapy.

Chemotherapy Anti-cancer drug usually given intravenously but sometimes by mouth. Chemo drugs are often given in combination for maximal effect, generally as repeated cycles or pulses of treatment on a regular three- or four-week basis, often to a total of six courses. There is now an enormous variety of these agents – new ones are appearing all the time.

Chemotherapy schedule A chemotherapy treatment plan generally employing agents from different categories to gain the maximum cell kill with the minimum of side-effects.

CIN Carcinoma-in-situ. Severe cellular changes in an organ, with a recognisable pre-malignant change. Important in cancer of the cervix, larynx, etc.

Clone A cluster of cells derived from a single 'stem' or 'progenitor' cell.

CLL Chronic lymphocytic leukaemia. A more slowly evolving type of leukaemia compared to ALL. Doesn't occur in childhood. May not require initial treatment at all – often relatively indolent.

CMF Standard drug regimen used in the treatment of breast cancer. Stands for the widely used three-drug combination cyclophosphamide, methodrexate and fluorouracil.

CML Chronic myeloid leukaemia. A form of leukaemia arising from the myeloid white cell line in the marrow. May be treated by simple tablet chemotherapy or interferon in its early stages but may progress to a more rapidly evolving form. Sometimes curable by bone marrow transplantation; also responsive to a new wonder-drug recently introduced, a tyrosine kinese inhibitor known as STI-571 (see page 213).

Colonoscopy Examination of the whole large bowel using fibre-optic methods.

Colorectal A term used to denote the colon and rectum, often regarded together as the key primary sites for carcinoma of the large bowel.

Contralateral primary Development of a new cancer on the opposite side. Particularly applies to breast and testicular cancers.

Conformal external beam irradiation Relatively new form of radiotherapy in which the beam is shaped to conform to the outline of the tumour, using computer-controlled lead mini-blocks. Allows for better shielding of the normal tissues surrounding the tumour, hence a safe increase in dose to the tumour itself.

Cryosurgery Treatment by freezing.

CT scan Computer tomography. Very common and informative type of scanning device, now widely available.

Cystectomy Surgical removal of the bladder.

Cystodiathermy Use of local heat application in the bladder to burn away a tumour.

Cytokines Biological substances, which are sometimes bone marrow stimulators or chemical messengers.

Cytotoxic therapy A treatment that is effective at killing cells. Chemotherapy is the major form of cytotoxic therapy.

Desquamation Skin damage, of the type characteristically caused by radiation. Divided into dry and moist (the latter more severe) but usually recovers completely.

Dysphagia Difficulty in swallowing.

Dysphasia Difficulty with speech.

Dysplasia Cellular change with an atypical, but not yet malignant, appearance.

Dyspnoea Shortness of breath.

Emetogenic treatment Treatment with an agent likely to cause nausea – e.g. some, *though not all*, types of chemo. Anti-nausea drugs are far more effective than in the past.

Endoscopy An internal inspection using a semi-rigid fibre-optic telescope. Widely used, e.g. for bronchus, stomach, head and neck areas.

Epidemiology Studies of different populations, often giving remarkable clues or insights into cancer causation and treatment response.

EUA Examination under anaesthesia.

Gastrostomy A specially positioned stomach tube for feeding purposes. Usually temporary.

Germ cell tumour See Teratoma.

Glioma The most common type of brain tumour.

GVHD Graft versus host disease. A condition in which the grafted or transplanted tissue attacks the patient, whose host defences have had to be deliberately reduced for the transplants to 'take' in the first place. May occur, for example, in cases of allogeneic bone marrow transplantation.

Haemoptysis Coughing up blood.

HCG Human chorionic gonadotrophin. A tumour marker substance made by certain types of malignant tissue – a rise may often denote testicular cancer. See also AFP – but the cell of origin is different.

Hemicolectomy A large bowel resection, in which approximately half the bowel is removed.

Hemiglossectomy Surgical removal of half of the tongue.

Hepatoma Primary cancer of the liver.

Hickman line A long, in-dwelling, hollow, small-bore, flexible, sterile plastic tube (cannula) entering the body via the skin (usually placed over the chest wall) but ending deep in the large veins close to the heart. Often used to deliver chemotherapy, blood transfusions and for taking blood samples. The tube may remain in place for months and makes the patient's life more comfortable over a lengthy treatment period.

Hormone therapy Several human tissues can produce hormones, e.g. ovary (oestrogen), testis (testosterone). Certain cancers, e.g. breast, prostate, often require these for their continued growth, so hormone antagonists, e.g. tamoxifen (predominantly an anti-oestrogen), can be very effective.

Hydrocephalus Swelling of the fluid-filled ventricles of the brain, often caused by an obstructive brain tumour or other 'space-occupying' lesion.

Hysterectomy Surgical removal of the uterus (womb). Often a curative procedure for cancers of the uterus and cervix.

Initiator The underlying or first event that destabilises the cell and mutates it in the direction of cancer growth.

Large-cell carcinomas Forms a group with squamous cell and adenocarcinoma, often considered jointly for treatment purposes, in the case of lung cancer.

Laryngectomy Surgical removal of the larynx (voice-box). Can be curative for laryngial cancer.

Laser surgery A form of treatment using an intense and pure light source of a particular wavelength. Extremely useful for certain cancers. Can unblock organs such as the oesophagus, allowing much improved nutrition during more definitive treatment, e.g. with radical chemo-radiation therapy.

Leiomyosarcoma A type of soft-tissue sarcoma, arising from smooth muscle.

Liposarcoma A type of soft-tissue sarcoma, arising from fatty tissue.

Lobectomy Removal of part of an organ, e.g. the lung or liver, leaving the remainder intact.

Lumpectomy Local excision of a primary tumour mass – widely used in breast cancer, allowing excellent preservation of the breast itself.

Lymphoedema Swelling of the arm from excess tissue fluid. Most common after treatment for breast cancer, in which axillary dissection and radiation to the area have both been necessary.

Lymphomas The general name for malignancies arising from lymph node tissues. Hodgkin's disease is one example but there are many others.

Mastectomy Surgical removal of the breast.

Medulloblastoma A form of paediatric brain tumour, arising from the hind-part (cerebellum) of the brain.

Metastasis (plural metastases) Secondary growth of cancer, often distant from the main site.

Mitotic rate The rate at which cells are actively dividing. Often increased well above normal in the case of cancer.

MRI scan Magnetic resonance imaging – a sophisticated form of scanning; safe and repeatable since it does not involve radiation exposure.

Myeloma A malignant bone-marrow disorder with many specific features. Responsive to chemotherapy.

Myelosuppression Bone marrow failure, leading to reduction in the blood count.

Nasopharynx Area directly behind the nose. An important primary site for cancer, very common in South East Asia.

Neoplastic growth Often used as a synonym for cancer or malignancy.

Nephrectomy Surgical removal of the kidney.

Neutropenia Suppression of the white cells, which are essential for defence against infection. Often the result of chemotherapy but usually only temporary.

Occult disease Not readily visible but detectable radiologically or by other means, e.g. a raised tumour marker in the blood.

Oesophagitis Inflammation of the oesophagus.

Oncogenes Genes that drive a cell towards malignancy.

Orchidectomy Surgical removal of the testicle.

Osteosarcoma One of the major varieties of primary malignant bone tumour, though as a group, these diseases are extremely uncommon.

Pap smear Cervical screening test.

Peripheral blood stem cell transplantation (PBSC) The patient's bone marrow is stimulated by low-dose chemotherapy and other biological agents to liberate early marrow precursor cells. These are collected, concentrated and returned to the patient, as support for high-dose chemotherapy.

Pleural effusion Collection of fluid (not always malignant but always suspicious) within the chest.

Pneumonectomy Surgical removal of the lung.

Primary site Initial site of origin of a cancer in the body.

Prognosis Likely outcome; general outlook.

Prostatectomy Surgical removal of the prostate.

PSA Prostate-specific antigen. A tumour marker specifically relating to prostate cancer. A good guide to response and prognosis.

Radiotherapy Major form of cancer treatment, often used as an adjunct to surgery or even as primary therapy in inoperable cases. Can be curative. Increasingly used to avoid the inevitable tissue destruction caused by surgery. In wide use since its initial discovery over 100 years ago by Röntgen and the Curies.

Retinoblastoma A rare childhood cancer affecting the eye.

Rhabdomyosarcoma A type of soft-tissue sarcoma, arising from striped muscle.

Sarcoma A primary cancer growth in soft tissue or occasionally bone. Surgery is generally the best treatment.

Secondary site Further development in the body of a cancer, distant from the primary site. See 'metastasis'.

Seminoma A type of testicular germ-cell tumour, often very responsive to treatment. Excellent cure rate.

Sigmoidoscopy Endoscopic inspection of the lower (sigmoid) part of the colon.

Small-cell cancer Type of lung cancer very closely associated with cigarette smoking – almost unknown in non-smokers. Characterised by early and widespread dissemination in the body. Initially highly responsive to chemotherapy.

Squamous carcinoma A major type of cancer, originating from a body surface, e.g. skin, bronchus, cervix, head-and-neck sites.

Systemic Whole-body, e.g. used for treatments such as chemotherapy, hormones, which circulate throughout the body.

Teletherapy Type of radiation therapy where the treatment is applied as one or more external beams. The most common type of radiotherapy.

Teratoma A group of testicular germ-cell tumours, highly responsive to chemotherapy and usually curable (95% of cases), even when the tumour has spread beyond the primary site in the testis.

TNM staging system A method for describing the extent of a tumour. 'T' stands for 'tumour', 'N' for 'nodes' and 'M' for 'metastasis'. The system allows for an accurate description of the tumour characteristics, often a good pointer towards prognosis (see page 27).

TUR Trans-urethral resection procedure.

Ultrasound scanning Simple, inexpensive and valuable type of scanning using a similar principle to radar, passing radiowaves through an organ, and picking up the pattern of activity.

USEFUL ADDRESSES

Please be aware that the contact details of the following organisations may change and that websites may be updated and developed. To the best of our knowledge, details were correct as we went to press.

GENERAL SERVICES

BBC Education
www.bbc.co.uk/health/cancer
Website offering information about cancer in general: advice on treatment and seeking professional help, complementary medicine, a reading list and interviews with celebrities.

Bristol Cancer Help Centre
Grove House, Cornwallis Grove,
Clifton, Bristol BS8 4PG
Helpline: 0117 980 9505
E-mail: info@bristolcancerhelp.org
www.bristolcancerhelp.org

Healing programmes that are complementary to medical treatment and deal with mind and body – aspects include counselling, meditation, nutrition, music, art therapy and visualisation.

CancerBACUP
3 Bath Place, Rivington Street,
London EC2A 3JR
Freephone Cancer Information Services:
0808 800 1234
Tel: 020 7696 9003
Fax: 020 7696 9002
Scotland: 0141 553 1553
www.cancerbacup.org.uk
Information, emotional support and practical advice by telephone and letter, from professional cancer nurses; free factsheets on cancer and treatment; local centres in Nottingham, Coventry, London and Glasgow.

Cancer Care Society
11 The Corn Market,
Romsey, Hampshire SO51 8GE
Tel: 01794 830 374 (Mon-Fri, 9am-5pm)
Fax: 01794 518 133
E-mail: info@cancercaresociety.org
www.cancercaresociety.org
Free confidential counselling, emotional support and practical help for all cancer patients; complementary therapies; information library; telephone link to others with cancer.

CancerHelp UK
Website: www.cancerhelp.org.uk
Free information service about cancer and cancer care for the general public; run by The Cancer Research Campaign (see opposite); extensive information on cancer and its prevention; also provides further reading and a contact list of useful organisations.

Cancerlink
c/o Macmillan Cancer Relief (see below)
Freephone Support Link: 0800 800
0000 (Mon, Wed, Fri, 10am-6pm)
E-mail: cancerlink@cancerlink.org.uk
www.cancerlink.org
*Free confidential support services for
people affected by cancer; provides
resources, consultancy and training for
cancer self-help and support groups;
nationwide.*

The Cancer Research Campaign (CRC)
10 Cambridge Terrace, London NW1 4JL
Tel: 020 7224 1333
Fax: 020 7487 4310
Web: www.crc.org.uk
*National charity founded in 1923 to
research the causes of cancer, find ways
of preventing it, develop new treatments
and ensure that those treatments reach
patients within the UK and throughout
the world; supported by volunteer work
and nationwide fundraising events.
(see below for branches). Also runs
www.cancerhelp.org.uk (see opposite).*

CRC – Central & Anglia
Regional Director: Elizabeth Taylor
Mardall House, 9-11 Vaughan Road,
Harpenden, Hertfordshire AL5 4HU
Tel: 01582 764 832
Fax: 01582 764 474
E-mail: central&anglia@crc.org.uk

CRC – London & South East
Acting Regional Director: Helen Wright
89 Albert Embankment,
London SE1 7TP
Tel: 020 7820 6900
Fax: 020 7820 6990
E-mail: london&southeast@crc.org.uk

CRC – North West
Regional Director: Joanna Lavelle
Furness House, Furness Quay,
Salford Quays, Manchester M5 2XA
Tel: 0161 772 5555
Fax: 0161 772 5550
E-mail: northwest@crc.org.uk

CRC – South West
Regional Director: Claudia McVie
The Old Chapel Building,
Gloucester Road, Horfield,
Bristol BS7 0BJ
Tel: 0117 952 5464
Fax: 0117 952 5310
E-mail: southwest@crc.org.uk

CRC – Yorkshire & North East
Regional Director: Pat Bradley
The Manor House, 11-13 North Street,
Wetherby, North Yorkshire LS22 6NU
Tel: 01937 588 855
Fax: 01937 588 866
E-mail: yorks&northeast@crc.org.uk

See also Northern Ireland, Scotland and
Wales.

Cancer Resource Centre
PO Box 17, 20-22 York Road,
London SW11 3QE
Tel: 020 7924 3924
Fax: 020 7978 6505
E-mail:
info@cancer-resource-centre.org.uk
www.cancer-resource.org.uk
*Charity providing support, information
and complementary therapies for cancer
patients, families, friends and health
professionals; home-visiting service.*

CancerWEB
The Gray Cancer Institute
PO Box 100, Mount Vernon Hospital
Northwood, Middlesex HA6 2JR
Tel: 01923 828 611
E-mail: cancerweb@www.graylab.ac.uk
www.graylab.ac.uk/cancerweb.html
*Website offering extensive cancer
information on causes, prevention,
diagnosis and treatment; online medical
dictionary; links to health databases.*

CHAI – Lifeline Cancer Support and
Centre for Health
Norwood House,
Harmony Way, off Victoria Road,
London NW4 2BZ
Helpline: 020 8202 4567
E-mail: info@chai-lifeline.org.uk
www.chai-lifeline.org.uk
*Emotional support for Jewish cancer
patients, their families and friends, via
telephone, at home or in hospital;
complementary therapies; weekly
support group; monthly coffee mornings.*

The Compassionate Friends
53 North Street, Bristol BS3 1EN
Helpline: 0117 953 9639
www.tcf.org.uk
*An open self-help group of bereaved
parents (befriending rather than
counselling); provides newsletter and a
range of information leaflets; library
postal service.*

Gilda's Club London
14 Bury Place, London WC1A 2JL
Tel: 020 7440 9150
Fax: 020 7440 9151
www.gildas.org
*Services include support and networking
groups, workshops and lectures,
children's club and social events.*

Imperial Cancer Research Fund –
Cancer Information Service
61 Lincoln's Inn Fields,
London WC2A 3PX
Tel (Information and Support Services):
020 7269 3662.
E-mail: cancer.info@icrf.icnet.uk
www.imperialcancer.co.uk
*Employs over 1,000 doctors to research
the causes of cancer and its prevention,
and develop new treatments; website
provides information on cancer.*

Macmillan Cancer Relief (MCR)
89 Albert Embankment,
London SE1 7UQ
*UK-wide charity dedicated to the
treatment and care of cancer patients
and their families; specialist Macmillan
nurses and doctors; buildings for cancer
treatment and care; grants for patients
in financial difficulties.*

MCR – Central England
Fernhill Court,
Balsall Street, Balsall Common,
Coventry, West Midlands CV7 7FR
Tel: 01676 535452
Fax: 01676 535450

MCR – London, Anglia and South East
3 Angel Walk,
Hammersmith, London W6 9HX
Tel: 020 8563 9800
Fax: 020 8563 9640

MCR – Northern England
Hamilton House, 3 Fawcett Street,
York YO10 4AH
Tel: 01904 651700
Fax: 01904 654668

MCR – South West England
6 Regents Court, South Way,
Andover, Hampshire SP10 5NX
Tel: 01264 343800
Fax: 01264 343806

See also Northern Ireland, Scotland and
Wales.

Marie Curie Cancer Care
89 Albert Embankment,
London SE1 7TP
Tel: 020 7599 7729
Fax: 020 7599 7708
Freephone: 0800 716 146
E-mail: info@mariecurie.org.uk
www.mariecurie.org.uk
*Eleven hospice centres for cancer
patients throughout the UK;
community nursing service for cancer
patients and their carers at home (free
of charge to cancer patients).*

National Cancer Alliance
PO Box 579, Oxford OX4 1LB
Tel: 01865 793566
Fax: 01865 251 050
E-mail:
nationalcanceralliance@btinternet.com
www.nationalcanceralliance.co.uk
*Represents the interests of patients and
cancer campaigns, to ensure high
standards of treatment and care;
provides advice to the Department of
Health and NHS; publications available.*

New Approaches to Cancer
St Peter's Hospital, Guildford Road,
Chertsey, Surrey KT16 0PZ
Freephone: 0800 389 2662
Tel: 01932 879 882
E-mail: help@anac.org.uk
Fax: 01932 874 349
www.anac.org.uk
*Promotes the positive benefits of
complementary therapies and holistic
treatment for cancer patients.*

The Richard Dimbleby Cancer
Information & Support Service
2nd Floor, Lambeth Wing,
St Thomas' Hospital,
Lambeth Palace Rd, London SE1 7EH
Helpline: 020 7960 5682
Tel: 020 7960 5689
Fax: 020 7960 5687
E-mail:
joanne.jackson@gstt.sthames.nhs.uk;
karen.martin@gstt.sthames.nhs.uk
*Information and support for cancer
patients, their friends, families and the
health professionals who look after
them; cancer information library;
complementary therapies.*

NORTHERN IRELAND
Action Cancer
1 Marlborough Park, Belfast BT9 6XS

Helpline: 028 9024 4200
Tel: 028 9080 3344
Fax: 028 9080 3356
E-mail: supportservices@actioncancer.org
Website: www.actioncancer.org
*Full-time screening clinics for breast
and cervical cancer; information, advice
and evening clinics for prostate and
testicular cancers; mobile service for
people in rural communities;
information and counselling service.*

Cancer Research Campaign
Regional Director: Bill McKinley
Unit 1, The Pavilions, Kinnegar Drive,
Holywood, Co. Down BT18 9JQ
Tel: 01232 426 667
Fax: 01232 424 717
E-mail: northernireland@crc.org.uk

Macmillan Cancer Relief
Hamilton House, 82 Eglantine Avenue,
Belfast BT9 6EU
Tel: 01232 661 166
Fax: 01232 661 663

The Ulster Cancer Foundation
40-42 Eglantine Avenue, Belfast BT9 6DX
Cancer Helpline: 0800 783 3339 (Mon-
Fri, 9am-5pm)
*Information helpline for patients and
their families; counselling by personal
appointment; rehabilitation services.*

SCOTLAND
Macmillan Cancer Relief
9 Castle Terrace, Edinburgh EH1 2DP
Tel: 0131 229 3276
Fax: 0131 228 6710

CLAN - Cancer Link Aberdeen & North
Cancer Support Centre
CLAN House,
Carline Place, Aberdeen AB25 2TH
Freephone: 0800 783 7922
Tel: 01224 647000
E-mail: clan@btinternet
*Support, information and
complementary therapy for people
affected by cancer; residential
accommodation available.*

Cancer Research Campaign
Regional Director: Bill McKinlay
Federation House, 222 Queensferry Rd,
Edinburgh EH4 2BN
Tel: 0131 343 1344
Fax: 0131 343 6812
E-mail: scotland@crc.org.uk

Tak Tent Cancer Support
Flat 5, 30 Shelley Court,
Gartnavel Complex, Glasgow G12 07N
Helpline: 0141 211 1932
Fax: 0141 211 3988
www.taktent.org.uk
*Support and information for patients,
relatives, friends and helpers; network of
monthly support groups across Scotland.*

WALES
Macmillan Cancer Relief
Lloyds Bank Chambers,
33 High Street, Cowbridge,
South Glamorgan CF71 7AE
Tel: 01446 775 679
Fax: 01466 775 085

Cancer Research Campaign
Regional Director: Claudia McVie
Hamilton Court,
373 Cowbridge Road East,
Canton, Cardiff CF5 1JF
Tel: 01222 224 386
Fax: 01222 667 120
E-mail: wales@crc.org.uk

Tenovus Cancer Information Service
43 The Parade, Cardiff CF24 3AB
Freephone Helpline: 0808 808 1010
(Mon-Fri, 9am-4.30pm; answerphone
service on Wed pm and weekends)
Tel: 02920 482 000
E-mail: tciccancer@aol.com
www.tenovus.org.uk
*Emotional support and information on
cancer for patients and their families;
Freephone Helpline staffed by
experienced cancer trained nurses,
counsellors and a social worker; Drop-In
Centre for one-to-one counselling.*

BLADDER CANCER
Urostomy Association
Buckland, Beaumont Park,
Danbury, Essex CM3 4DE
Tel: 01245 224 294
Fax: 01245 227 569
www.uagbi.org
*Assistance for urostomy patients:
information service; help and advice on
post-treatment matters - using
everyday appliances, work situations
and relationships.*

BREAST CANCER
Breast Cancer Care
Kiln House, 210 New Kings Road,
London SW6 4NZ

Tel: 020 7384 2984
Fax: 020 7384 3387
Nationwide Freeline: 0808 800 6000
(10am–5pm, Monday to Friday)
Scottish Information Line: 0141 221 9499
E-mail: bcc@breastcancercare.org.uk
www.breastcancercare.org.uk
*Booklets, leaflets and tapes; prosthesis
fitting service; free helpline; one-to-one
emotional support from volunteers with
experience of breast cancer.*

Breast Care Campaign
Blythe Hall, 100 Blythe Road,
London W14 0HB
Tel: 020 7371 1510
Fax: 020 7371 4598
www.breastcare.co.uk
*Supplies fully referenced breast
bulletins, breast health information
leaflets and a bi-annual newsletter;
website of useful information.*

The Breast Clinic
www.thebreastclinic.com
*Website offering extensive information
on breast cancer; on-line discussion
forum; links to other useful websites.*

The London Haven
Effie Road, London SW6 1TB
The Haven Helpline: 08707 272 273
Services Information: 020 7384 0099
Admin. tel: 020 7384 0000
Fax: 020 7384 0002
E-mail: info@thehaventrust.org.uk
Website: www.thehaventrust.org.uk
*National support and information
helpline; free services for patients and
their families including breast care
nurse; lymphoedema service;
complementary therapies, counselling
and support services.*

Group for Women with Secondary
Breast Cancer
c/o Rosemary Burch,
Breast Care Counsellor,
St Thomas' Hospital,
Lambeth Palace Road, London SE1 7EH
Tel: 020 7928 9292 (ext.3864)
*Twice-monthly support group for
women with secondary breast cancer –
open to women across central London.*

CHILDREN
CLIC – Cancer and Leukaemia in
Childhood
Abbey Wood, Bristol B34 7JU

Telephone: 0117 311 2600
Fax: 0117 311 2649
E-mail: clic@clic-charity.demon.co.uk
www.clic.uk.com
*Support for young people (under 21
years of age) with any form of cancer or
leukaemia, and their families; provides
free accommodation adjacent to
paediatric oncology units, and a home
care nursing team; cash grants for any
special need.*

Captain Chemo
E-mail:
captainchemo@royalmarsden.org
www.royalmarsden.org/captchemo/
*Interactive website for children
providing information on the effects of
chemotherapy through a cartoon
character, Captain Chemo.*

Help Adolescents with Cancer
1st Floor, Post Office Building,
338 Hollinwood Avenue,
New Moston, Manchester M40 0JB
Tel: 0161 688 6244
Mobile: 0468 474 999
www.mwmsites.com/hawc
*National charity offering counselling,
group meetings and support for families
and siblings; annual 10-day workshop
for teenage patients.*

Sargent Cancer Care for Children
Griffin House, 161 Hammersmith Road,
London W6 8SG
Tel: 020 8752 2800
Fax: 020 8752 2806
E-mail: care@sargent.org
www.sargent.org
*Support for cancer patients under the
age of 21 (and their families), at home
and in hospital; counselling and advice;
financial assistance with clothing,
travel, fuel bills, etc.; short breaks,
workshops and vocational training.*

Christian Lewis Trust
62 Walters Road, Swansea,
West Glamorgan SA1 4PT
Freefone: 0800 303 031
Tel: 01792 480 500
Fax: 01792 480 700
E-mail: clt@aol.com
*Care for children with cancer and their
families; national helpline; welfare
grants, respite care, local support
groups, health education, care nurses,
social workers. and play therapists.*

COLORECTAL CANCER
British Colostomy Association
15 Station Road,
Reading, Berkshire RG1 1LG
Tel: 0118 939 1537
Fax: 0118 956 9095
E-mail: sue@bcass.org.uk
Freefone: 0800 328 4257
www.bcass.org.uk
*Emotional support and non-medical
help and advice; advisory booklet,
leaflets and twice-yearly newsletter;
visits to homes and hospitals available.*

Colon Cancer Concern
9 Rickett Street, London SW6 1RU
Infoline: 020 7381 9711 (10am–4pm)
E-mail: help@coloncancer.org.uk
Website: www.coloncancer.org.uk
*Conducts clinical trials to develop new
treatments for colorectal and secondary
liver cancer; Infoline for advice on
symptoms, tests, treatments and
keeping healthy.*

HEAD CANCERS
Brain Tumour Foundation
PO Box 162,
New Malden, Surrey KT3 3YN
Tel/Fax: 020 8336 2020
E-mail: btf.uk@virgin.net

British Brain and Spine Foundation
7 Winchester House, Cranmer Road,
Kennington Park, London SW9 6EJ
Brain and Spine Helpline: 0808 808
1000
Tel: 020 7793 5900
Fax: 020 7793 5939
E-mail: info@bbsf.org.uk
www.bbsf.org.uk
*Free telephone helpline; website
providing information via downloadable
books; personal accounts written by
patients.*

Changing Faces
1–2 Junction Mews, London W2 1PN
Tel: 020 7706 4232
Fax: 020 7706 4234
E-mail: info@changingfaces.co.uk
www.changingfaces.co.uk
*Provides support, either face-to-face, via
phone or letter; workshops; contact with
fellow cancer patients; self-help booklets
and videos on coping strategies and
communication skills; advice on
employment concerns, and making
medical and surgical treatment decisions.*

Let's Face It
14 Fallowfield,
Yateley, Hampshire GU17 7LW
Tel: 01252 879 630
Fax: 01252 872633
www.personal.u-net.com/~lfi/
Website for people of any age coping with facial disfigurement; links for people with similar experiences; contact by telephone and letter; meetings for self-help and social contact.

KIDNEY CANCER
Kidney Cancer UK
Tel: 024 7647 0584 (Keith Taylor)
E-mail: dick@mailbox.co.uk (Dick Williams)
www.kcuk.org
Support for kidney cancer patients and their carers; network of support groups; online website discussion group; twice-monthly newsletter and quarterly meetings.

LEUKAEMIA
The Leukaemia Care Society
2 Shrubbery Avenue,
Worcester WR1 1QH
Helpline: 0345 673203
Tel: 01905 330 003
Fax: 01905 330 0901
E-mail: enquiries@leukaemiacare.org.uk
www.leukaemiacare.org
Promotes the welfare of people with leukaemia and allied blood disorders; provides assistance for their families; offers family caravan holidays, friendship and support; limited financial assistance; free membership, newsletter and publications.

LYMPHOMA (HODGKIN'S AND NON-HODGKIN'S) AND LYMPHOEDEMA
Lymphoma Association
PO Box 386, Aylesbury, Bucks HP20 2GA
Freephone Helpline: 0808 808 5555
Admin tel: 01296 619 400
www.lymphoma.org.uk/support
Provides a range of downloadable information booklets and fact files; freephone helpline providing information and emotional support from trained staff; postal library service.

Lymphoma Resource Pages
www.lymphomainfo.net
Website offering extensive information on lymphomas and links to other useful websites.

Lymphoedema Support Network
St Luke's Crypt, Sydney Street,
London SW3 6NH
Information/Helpline: 020 7351 4480
Tel: 020 7351 4480
Fax: 020 7349 9809
E-mail: adminlsn@lymphoedema.freeserve.co.uk
www.lymphoedema.org/lsn/
Information and emotional support for patients with lymphoedema; quarterly newsletter; leaflets, factsheets and a video on breathing exercises.

LUNG CANCER
The Roy Castle Lung Cancer Foundation
200 London Road, Liverpool L3 9TA
Freefone: 0800 358 7200
Tel: 0151 794 8800
Fax: 0151 794 8888
www.roycastle.org
Website information, help and advice on lung cancer; patient support network; support nurses; community-based 'stop smoking' group; anti-tobacco campaign.

MELANOMA
Wessex Cancer Trust
Helpline: 01722 415071
www.wessexcancer.org
Telephone helpline; extensive cancer information and the latest cancer news; discussion pages.

MYELOMA
International Myeloma Foundation (UK)
9 Gayfield Square, Edinburgh EH1 3NT
Freephone: 0800 980 3332
Tel: 0131 557 3332
Fax: 0131 556 9720
E-mail: theimf@myeloma.org.uk
www.myeloma.org.uk
Free helpline; free IMF information pack; patient and family support network; website with a range of information on myeloma.

NEUROBLASTOMA
The Neuroblastoma Society
Alderwood, 9 Dominic Court,
Beaulieu Drive,
Waltham Abbey, Essex EN9 1JT
Tel: 01992 719696
Information and advice by telephone or letter for patients, their friends and families; contact with others who have experienced the illness in the family (where possible).

ORAL CANCERS
Oesophageal Patients' Association
16 Whitefields Crescent,
Solihull, West Midlands B91 3NU
Tel: 0121 704 9860
Provides leaflets, telephone advice and support before and during treatment; visits (where possible) by former patients to people with oesophageal cancer.

National Association of Laryngectomee Clubs
Ground Floor, 6 Rickett Street,
Fulham, London SW6 1RU
Tel: 020 7381 9993
Promotes the welfare of laryngectomees; support for the formation of clubs for rehabilitation assistance through speech therapy, social support and monthly meetings; advice on speech aids and medical supplies; referral service available.

OVARIAN CANCER
Ovacome
St Bartholomew's Hospital,
West Smithfield, London EC1A 7BE
Fone Friends: 07071 781 861
E-mail: internetfriends@ovacome.org.uk
www.dspace.dial.pipex.com/ovacome
Nationwide support group for ovarian cancer patients, their families, friends, carers and health professionals; links to other patients via the Fone Friends telephone network; information on treatments, screening and research.

PROSTATE AND TESTICULAR CANCER
Prostate Cancer Charity
3 Angel Walk,
Hammersmith, London W6 9HX
Helpline: 0845 300 8383
Admin tel: 020 8222 7622
Fax: 020 8222 7639
E-mail: info@prostate-cancer.org.uk
www.prostate-cancer.org.uk
Free information leaflets; telephone helpline staffed by counsellors; network of self-help groups.

Testicular Cancer Support
14 Blighmont Crescent, Millbrook,
Southampton, Hampshire SO15 8RH
Tel: 023 8077 5611
Voluntary group offering mutual support and self-help for men with testicular cancer.

RETINOBLASTOMA
Retinoblastoma Society
St Bartholomew's Hospital,
West Smithfield,
London EC1A 7BE
Tel: 020 7600 3309
Fax: 020 7600 8579
E-mail: rbinfo@rbsociety.org.uk
www.rbsociety.org.uk
*Information for families and
professionals on treatment; links
families of cancer patients in the same
geographical area; promotes and funds
research.*

HELP FOR WOMEN
Women's Nationwide Cancer Campaign
1st Floor, Charity House,
14-15 Perseverance Works,
London E2 8DD
Tel: 020 7729 4688
Fax: 020 7613 0771
E-mail: admin@wncc.org.uk
www.wnccc.org.uk
*Health education publications and
videos on cancer prevention and
screening; seminars and meetings
around the UK on issues surrounding
screening.*

Hysterectomy Support Network
3 Lynne Close, Green Street Green,
Orpington, Kent BR6 6BS
*Refers women, their families or partners
to former patients living locally –
encouragement, advice and support
through sharing of experiences and
information; booklet and other
information on local support groups;
contact by letter or group meetings.*

OTHER USEFUL ADDRESSES
British Acupuncture Council
63 Jeddo Road, London W12 9HQ
Tel: 020 8735 0400
Fax: 020 8735 0404
E-mail: info@acupuncture.org.uk
www.acupuncture.org.uk
*National organisation supplying a list of
local acupuncture practitioners.*

British Association for Counselling
1 Regent Place,
Rugby, Warwickshire CV21 2PJ
Tel: 0870 443 5252
Fax: 0870 443 5160
E-mail: bac@bac.co.uk
www.bac.co.uk
Information on training as a counsellor

*and on local counselling services;
support and protection for members of
the public seeking counselling.*

British Red Cross Society
9 Grosvenor Crescent,
London SW1X 7EJ
Tel: 020 7235 5454
Fax: 020 245 6315
E-mail: IWD@redcross.org.uk
www.redcross.org.uk
*Offers a range of services, including
short-term loan of medical equipment
(e.g. a wheelchair); Home from Hospital
service providing help for people arriving
home after treatment as an in-patient;
therapeutic care service.*

Carers National Association
20-25 Glasshouse Yard, London EC1A 4JT
Tel: 020 7490 8818
Fax: 020 7490 8824
Carers' Line: 0808 808 7777
www.carersuk.demon.co.uk
*Information and support for people
caring for relatives and friends; free
telephone line; a range of free leaflets
and information sheets.*

Crossroads – Caring for Carers
10 Regent Place,
Rugby, Warwickshire CV21 2PN
Helpline: 0500 179 546
Tel: 01788 573 653
Fax: 01788 565 498

Cruse Bereavement Care
126 Sheen Road, Richmond, Surrey
TW9 1UR
Helpline: 020 8332 7227 (Mon-Fri,
9.30am-5pm)
Counselling Line: 0345 585 565
Tel: 020 8940 4818
Fax: 020 8940 7638
Scotland: 0131 551 1511
*Free help to all bereaved people through
194 local branches; group counselling
providing social contact and practical
advice; free list of related publications
and newsletter.*

Courage UK
24 Lockett Gardens, Trinity,
Salford, Greater Manchester M3 6BJ
Tel: 0161 839 2927
Fax: 0161 839 4256
*Support groups offering mutual support
for patients with radiotherapy injury –
mainly in the pelvic area.*

The Hospice Information Service
St Christopher's Hospice,
51-59 Lawrie Park Road,
Sydenham, London SE26 6DZ
Tel: 020 8778 9252
Fax: 020 8776 9345
E-mail: info@his2.freeserve.co.uk
www.hospiceinformation.co.uk
*Publishes palliative care factsheets and
a directory of hospice and palliative care
services, hospices and home care teams.*

Institute for Complementary Medicine
PO Box 194, London SE16 7QZ
Tel: 020 7237 5165
Fax: 020 7237 5175
E-mail: icm@icmedicine.co.uk
www.icmedicine.co.uk
*Information on qualified complementary
practitioners, complementary teaching
institutions and complementary
medicine.*

Institute of Family Therapy
24-32 Stephenson Way,
London NW1 2HX
Tel: 020 7391 9150
Fax: 020 7391 9169
E-mail:
clinical@instituteoffamilytherapy.org.uk
www.instituteoffamilytherapy.org.uk
*Registered charity for families
experiencing difficulties including family
illness, loss and bereavement.*

The Sue Ryder Foundation
Kings House, Kings St,
Sudbury, Suffolk CO10 2ED
Tel: 01787 314200
Fax: 01787 319 516
E-mail: chris@sueryder.com
www.sueryder.com
*Centres throughout the UK including
homes specialising in cancer care;
visiting home care nurses; advice,
bereavement counselling and respite care.*

Urostomy Association
Buckland, Beaumont Park,
Danbury, Essex CM3 4DE
Tel: 01245 224294
E-mail: ua@centraloffice.fsnet.co.uk
www.uagbi.org
*Assistance for urostomy patients before
and after surgery; counselling on
appliances, housing, work situations or
marital problems; branch and house
meetings arranged; hospital and home
visits by former patients on request.*

INDEX

ACKNOWLEDGEMENTS

The authors and publishers are extremely grateful to all the patients who have given permission for their stories and experiences of cancer treatment to be included in this book. Very special thanks are extended to the families of the patients featured in the BBC TV series who have sadly died since their interviews took place. Without exception, the patients were enthusiastic about being included in this book, and were pleased that they might be helping others by sharing their experiences.

Thanks also are due to the following for their kind permission to reproduce the photographs on these pages: page 7 Gary Lineker; page 38 Press Association; page 39 Dr Frances Calman; page 61 Macmillan Cancer Relief.

Some of the contents of this book is based on material previously published in Cancer: what every patient needs to know by Dr Jeffrey Tobias (Bloomsbury, 1995, revised 1999).